Cook Right 4 Your Type

Also by Dr. Peter J. D'Adamo
with Catherine Whitney

Eat Right 4 Your Type

DR. PETER J. D'ADAMO

WITH CATHERINE WHITNEY

G. P. PUTNAM'S SONS
NEW YORK

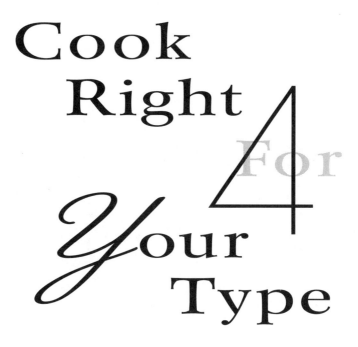

Cook Right 4 For Your Type

THE PRACTICAL KITCHEN COMPANION TO *EAT RIGHT 4 YOUR TYPE*

*Including More Than
200 Original Recipes,
as Well as Individualized
30-Day Meal Plans for
Staying Healthy, Living Longer,
and Achieving Your Ideal Weight*

G. P. Putnam's Sons
Publishers Since 1838
a member of Penguin Putnam Inc.
375 Hudson Street
New York, NY 10014

Library of Congress Cataloging-in-Publication Data

D'Adamo, Peter.
Cook right 4 your type : the practical kitchen companion
to eat right 4 your type, including more than 200 original recipes, as well as
individualized 30-day meal plans for staying healthy, living longer, and achieving
your ideal weight / by Peter J. D'Adamo, with Catherine Whitney.

p.   cm.
ISBN 0-399-14437-4
1. Blood groups.   2. Nutrition.   3. Cookery.
I. Whitney, Catherine (Catherine A.)   II. Title.
QP98.D327   1999   98-28749   CIP
613.2'6—dc21

Printed in the United States of America
5   7   9   10   8   6   4

TO CHRISTL AND DAD
WITH LOVE

Acknowledgments

IT IS MY GREAT PLEASURE TO BRING TO THE READERS OF *Eat Right 4 Your Type* this practical kitchen companion to help you more effectively incorporate the Blood Type Diet into your daily lives. There are many people to thank, as this was truly a group effort.

I am grateful to Putnam for its continuing support of my work; in particular, my editor, Amy Hertz (Type B), whose personal and professional commitment has helped make the Blood Type Diet an outstanding success. And to my dedicated literary agent, Janis Vallely (Type O), whose encouragement and guidance have made this book possible.

Special thanks to all the people who worked so hard to make *Cook Right 4 Your Type* happen:

Catherine Whitney (Type O), my writer, who organized and crafted the text, along with her team, Martha Mosko D'Adamo (Type O) and Paul Krafin (Type A). The combination of solid writing, thorough research, and attention to detail has produced a truly valuable resource.

Our chefs, Martine Lloyd Warner (Type O) and Gabrielle Lloyd Sindorf (Type O), who contributed their skill and imagination to the development of the wonderful recipes in this book.

Jane Dystel (Type B), Catherine's literary agent, who has lent valuable advice at every stage.

John Finley, for his beautifully designed illustrations.

Sally Cardy Mosko (Type A) for her easy-to-read charts.

The "cyber cooks" who donated their favorite recipes, and my "cyber friends," Heidi Merritt (Type O) and Steve Shapiro (Type O), who have been such a great help to me on the Web site, www.dadamo.com.

Cheryl Miller (Type O) for her always helpful ideas and recipe advice. Janet Schuler (Type O) for her secretarial support.

Thanks, too, to Scott Carlson (Type A), my assistant, who makes the office run so smoothly; Carolyn Knight, R.N. (Type A), my invaluable nurse; and my wonderful, supportive staff: Wendy Carlson (Type A), Melissa Danelowski (Type O) and Richard Tuzzio (Type A).

Special thanks to the professionals who have given their support to this work, in particular Michael Finney (Type A), Jay Fiano (Type B), Michael Schacter, M.D. (Type O), Ronald Hoffman, M.D. (Type O), Joseph Pizzorno, N.D. (Type A), Thomas Kruzel, N.D. (Type B), William Mitchell, N.D. (Type O), and Jeffrey Bland, Ph.D. (Type O). It has been a special privilege to work closely with a very talented clinician, Gregory Kelly, N.D. (Type A), whose integrity, professionalism, and editing skills have greatly contributed to the veracity of this work.

I am also grateful to the hundreds of thousands of readers who have spread the word about the Blood Type Diet and who have shared their successes and difficulties, helped perfect the science, and contributed countless valuable suggestions. Every day I am encouraged by the level of dialogue and the excitement that comes through the mail and on the Web site.

I am fortunate to have the never-failing support and encouragement of my family: Christl (Type B) and Dad (Type A); my brother, James D'Adamo (Type A), and his fiancée, Ann (Type A); and my sister, Michele (Type AB). A special acknowledgment to my mother-in-law, Mary Mosko (Type O), for her never-failing faith and courage.

Finally, I am enchanted every day by the spirit of my young daughters, Claudia (Type A) and Emily (Type A) and blessed by the love and kindness of my wife, Martha (Type O).

Contents

The Eat Right Road Map

The Blood Type Diet

A Celebration of Individuality

*I*N THE TWO YEARS SINCE THE PUBLICATION OF *EAT Right 4 Your Type,* I have communicated with hundreds of thousands of people during media appearances, on the Web, over the phone, by mail, at lectures, and in my office. Many of them have been curious, a few skeptical, and some true believers in the Blood Type Diet. On my Web site, people share, with touching detail, their long efforts to find a key to a chronic illness or a battle with obesity. Their stories have many common elements, but at the core they are utterly unique and individual—just like the people themselves. They have helped me appreciate more than ever before the countless variations among humans.

Does the Blood Type Diet work? What I have learned from collecting thousands of certified medical results from readers and patients is that it works for nine out of ten people and that the more severe the problem, the faster it works. But the real question each person needs to ask is, "Does it work for me?" It is not as important to have a theory that works for everybody in a generic way as it is to have a theory that takes into account individual variations.

The Blood Type Diet is really about the expression of individuality. Properly understood, individuality becomes a powerful friend, allowing a deeper grasp of the whys and wherefores of a given medical or health condition. If individual variations are ignored or downplayed, they become roadblocks that devalue the very best science has to offer. So when you hear or read about a new scientific finding, always ask the question, "Are they talking about me?"

How can you find out whether or not the Blood Type Diet is right for you? First, you must be willing to change your mind-set about food. We have all been conditioned to view food as one thing and medicine another. We are rarely asked to consider the multifaceted ways in which the food we eat affects every cell in our bodies. Because of this, it can be uncomfortable to grapple with new ideas, such as those presented in the Blood Type Diet. But when you consider that most of our current knowledge about human nutrition has been acquired in this century, you can see that we are only just beginning to understand the effect of foods on our bodily systems.

Cook Right 4 Your Type has been developed in response to the clamor for practical ways to use the Blood Type Diet in everyday life. View it as a guide to help you put the blood type recommendations into practice, so that you can fully experience the health benefits of eating the foods that are right for you.

You will find no absolutes in this book. The Blood Type Diet has never been about rigid rules and regulations. Nor is it about superimposing an artificial set of values on the way you already live. Eating right for your blood type simply means following the ancient codes that are still imprinted in every cell of your body. Think of it as one of the ways you can celebrate the miracle of human individuality.

The Genetic Fingerprint

Why Your Blood Type Matters

*T*HE SCIENCE OF BLOOD TYPE HAS BEEN EVOLVING ever since the beginning of known human history. It is the science of individuality—an acknowledgment that each of us has a genetic fingerprint located in the cells of our bodies.

Before you begin using *Cook Right 4 Your Type*, you need to understand the reason why your blood type can make such a crucial difference in how you live and what you eat. Blood type is not a neutral factor. Rather, it behaves as the control valve of your immune and digestive systems, a biologic watchdog that enhances your body's ability to survive and thrive.

My first book, *Eat Right 4 Your Type*, fully explains the mechanism by which your blood type responds to the food you eat—either for good or for ill. It details the scientific and anthropological reasons for the four distinct blood types. I urge you to read it as both an aid and an introduction to *Cook Right 4 Your Type*. The following is a brief summary of that information.

The Key to Survival

ALMOST EVERYONE, including physicians, considers the importance of blood type only in relation to transfusions. The gross limitations imposed by such a narrow view become readily apparent when you consider the central role blood type has played in the survival of the human race. Consider this: Were it not for the unique adaptations that have taken place within the blood, the human race would not have been able to survive.

Each of the four blood types evolved in response to both the physiologic development of the species and changing climatic conditions over the eons since humankind first trod the Earth. This is the vital clue to the importance of blood type. The adaptations that occurred in the course of evolution not only strengthened our immune systems against new bacterial, viral, and environmental assailants, but at the same time permitted our vulnerable digestive systems to adapt to a wide range of unfamiliar foods.

Type O

The first known blood type was Type O, which dates as far back as the ascendence of the Cro-Magnons and remains today as the most common blood type worldwide. Type O, which we call "the hunter," has a strong and ornery immune system and a hearty digestive system. The strength of the Type O immune and digestive systems ensured early survival because meat was the primary food source. The Type O has an extraordinarily high stomach-acid content, capable of drawing the most nutrients from meat and efficiently assimilating such a protein-heavy balance of foods.

You might say that Type Os were the first humans to eat on the run. They hunted where they were led by their prey, killed it, consumed it, and moved on. But over time, the vast herds of available game began at last to thin. As the human race continued to evolve, the desire for survival forced many to learn the skills of growing and preserving a food supply that would protect against famine. This new system demanded that humans remain in one favorable geographic area and create settled cooperative societies that would devote themselves to sustaining the agrarian cycle. Living in communities not only demanded new social skills, it also gave rise to new diseases.

Type A

Type A, which began to gain prominence between 25,000 and 15,000 B.C., differentiated its immune system from that of Type O to fight off infections and bacteria that were decimating the collectives, while the Type A digestive system adapted to a diet that was able to meet the body's need for proteins derived primarily from plants and grains. At the same time, lakes, rivers, and seas provided a bounty of fish that incorporated yet another abundant protein source into the human diet. We refer to these new Type As as "the cultivators."

Type B

Type B began appearing between 15,000 and 10,000 B.C., as the growing tide of humanity spread beyond the range of the first Type O hunters and moved out from the settled agrarian Type A communities—one reason we call Type B "the nomads." Century after century, enormous tribes traveled across the endless landscapes of a still primitive and ever-changing world, surviving on the meat and dairy of the cattle, goats, and sheep they herded as well as on whatever they scavenged along the way. Because Type B incorporated so many of the immune- and digestive-system characteristics of Type O and Type A, they developed a system more balanced and tolerant than that of either of the previous types.

Type AB

For most of our history there have been three blood types, and then, approximately ten to fifteen centuries ago, Type AB, still very rare, emerged. We often call Type AB "the enigma," because it isn't entirely clear what stimulated this latest blood type adaptation. Perhaps the full evolution of Type AB is yet to come. What we do know is that it combines most of the strengths and weaknesses of both Type A and Type B. The Type AB immune and digestive system is more complex and quirky than any of the others, which is both good and bad. The good resides in its wide range of immune and digestive responses; the bad in its incorporation of the frailties and vulnerabilities of both Type A and Type B.

The Science of Blood

So WHAT DOES blood type actually do in the body that makes its impact so significant? Each blood type is named for its biochemical differences—specifically, its antigens.

Antigens are chemical markers that are found on the cells of our bodies. Antigens spark the production of antibodies. Each blood type possesses a different antigen with its own special chemical structure.

| | YOU HAVE THIS ANTIGEN(S) |
IF YOU ARE	ON YOUR CELLS
BLOOD TYPE O	NO ANTIGENS
BLOOD TYPE A	A
BLOOD TYPE B	B
BLOOD TYPE AB	A and B

Imagine the chemical structure of our blood types as antennae of sorts, projecting outward from the surface of our cells into deep space. These antennae are made up of long chains of a repeating sugar called *fucose*. Fucose forms the simplest of the blood types, Blood Type O. One sugar equals Type O.

Blood Type A cells looks just like Type O cells, except a Type A cell has two antennae coming out of it. So Type A is formed when the O antigen, made of fucose, plus another sugar, called N-acetyl-galactosamine, are combined. These two sugars equal Type A.

Blood Type B cells look just like Type A cells. Type B also has two antennae. The difference is that the second antenna of Type B is made of a different kind of sugar than that of Type A. Type B is comprised of the O antigen sugar fucose, plus another sugar, called D-galactose. So two *other* sugars equal Type B.

Blood Type AB cells have three antennae radiating out of them. Type AB contains the Type O antigen, fucose, as well as the Type A sugar, N-acetyl-galactosamine, and the Type B sugar, D-galactose. In this case, the three sugars that singularly or in combination compose the other three blood types equal Type AB.

The Blood Type–Diet Connection

How DOES the composition of the sugars that make up the blood types relate to what you eat? A chemical reaction occurs between your blood and the foods you consume. We know this because of a factor called *lectins*. Lectins are abundant and diverse proteins found in foods. They have agglutinating—gluing or sticking—properties that affect your blood. When you eat a food containing protein lectins that are incompatible with your blood type antigen, the lectins target an organ and begin to agglutinate blood cells in that area. In effect, lectins gum up the works, interfering with digestion, insulin production, food metabolism, and hormonal balance.

Many people who first read of lectins in *Eat Right 4 Your Type* questioned me about why they'd never heard of them before.

Some were skeptical. Surely, they said, if lectins had ever been a real concern, physicians and nutritionists would have long ago brought their effects to light. Those skeptics were surprised when I informed them that hundreds of scientific papers have been written about the effects of lectins. The fact that they haven't had wider public exposure relegates lectins to the province of a well-kept secret. Apparently, *Eat Right 4 Your Type* was the first time that the results of the extensive scientific research had ever appeared in a mainstream publication.

Knowing about the potential danger of lectins does not mean that you should suddenly become fearful of every food you eat. After all, lectins are widely abundant and hard to avoid. The key is to avoid the lectins that agglutinate your blood type. For example, gluten, the most common lectin found in wheat, has a shape different from the lectin found in soy, and it attaches to a different combination of sugars. Gluten binds to the lining of the small intestine and can cause substantial inflammation and painful irritation in some blood types, particularly Type O. Chicken, on the other hand, which is fine for Type Os and Type As, contains a lectin in its muscle tissue that agglutinates Type B and Type AB blood cells.

What This Means for You

HERE'S THE BOTTOM LINE: We are predisposed to certain strengths and weaknesses according to our blood types. We can maximize our strengths and minimize our weaknesses by knowing what our bodies need and by feeding ourselves and our families accordingly.

The crux of *Eat Right 4 Your Type* resides in the fact that certain foods complement certain blood types. Other foods antagonize and debilitate particular blood types. By stressing the complementary foods and eliminating clearly antagonistic foods, you can promote the best possible balance for your immune and digestive systems. Most of your compatible foods correspond to

---

Do You Know Your Blood Type?

There are several ways to find out your blood type.

1. Donate blood. Also note that blood banks will often perform a blood type test for a fee, even if you don't wish to give blood.
2. Ask your doctor—but don't be surprised if he or she doesn't know. When blood is drawn for routine cholesterol screening or other factors, blood typing is not normally done unless it has been requested.
3. Refer to the appendices of this book to order an easy, accurate at-home blood type testing kit.

---

your blood type's evolutionary development. In other words, the foods that fit your blood type are often the very foods that were predominant at the time in history when your blood type first appeared. For example:

If you are Type O, you respond best to a high-protein diet, including meat, poultry, fish, and a variety of fruits and vegetables. Many grains, legumes, and dairy products are incompatible with your blood type.

If you are Type A, you thrive on a primarily vegetarian diet, including soy products, beans and legumes, grains, vegetables, and fruits, with small portions of fish.

If you are Type B, your optimal diet includes game meat like rabbit and venison as well as herd meats, such as lamb and mutton. However, Type B should avoid chicken. Unlike Type O and Type A, Type B benefits from a variety of dairy products. Some grains, beans, and legumes cause problems for Type B, but there is a wide selection of vegetables and fruits available. In almost every respect, the Type B Diet is the most varied.

If you are Type AB, your diet is more complex—a combination of Type A and Type B. Type AB can eat most of the foods that are good for these blood types, but must avoid or limit most of the foods that agglutinate them. The best diet for Type AB consists primarily of vegetarian fare, with modest supplements of meat and dairy.

In the following pages you will find detailed charts and information that will help you *Eat Right 4 Your Type*. That means emphasizing the foods you find on the Highly Beneficial lists, restricting the foods you should Avoid, and incorporating the wide range of Neutral foods in a balanced and healthy way. As hundreds of thousands of people have discovered, eating right for your blood type can produce extraordinary and almost immediate results in combating allergies or other chronic conditions. Following your Blood Type Diet can also result in immediate changes—weight loss, restoration of normal insulin production, cessation of troublesome digestive problems, and an increase in energy and stamina. The long-term benefits are even more meaningful. The Blood Type Diet can help you combat serious illnesses, such as cancer and cardiovascular disease, avoid common viruses and infections, eliminate the toxins and fats that contribute to obesity, and slow the process of cell deterioration that accompanies aging. And the best news of all is that you can achieve all of these benefits while enjoying a healthy, satisfying, and varied diet. *Cook Right 4 Your Type* will provide you with wonderful recipes, food preparation hints, nutritional tips, and menus that will show you how to start eating right for your type. Good living and good health are yours to enjoy.

The Key to Eating Right

HIGHLY BENEFICIAL foods act like medicine in your body.

NEUTRAL foods act like food in your body.

AVOID foods act like poison in your body.

THREE

Humanity's Cornucopia

What Nutrition Really Means

*C*ATCH AS CATCH CAN DESCRIBES THE ORIGINAL DIET of humankind perfectly. Early humans were essentially carnivorous scavengers. If we were able to catch it, we ate it. That is not to say that our early ancestors ate nothing but meat. Plant life has always been part of the human diet. Humans are essentially *omnivores* (meat and plant eaters) rather than *herbivores* (plant eaters) or *carnivores* (meat eaters). But we are omnivores with many variations. There are cultures whose primary source of food comes from animals, such as the traditional Inuits of the Arctic region and the Masai tribes of Africa. Other cultures, such as the Bantus of Africa, are herbivores, and live as vegetarians. These seeming extremes are in perfect sync with our work on blood type. The carnivorous Inuits and Masai have large numbers of Type Os in their populations, while the effects of Type A development can be seen in the vegan Bantus in such strength that they have a blood subtype named for them—Type A-Bantu.

When we look at the effects of food on blood type in our ancestors, the picture is relatively simple. However, in modern times, we have complicated the picture, sometimes with disastrous consequences. Advances in agricultural methods and processing techniques began to strip foodstuffs of their essential ingredients and further remove them from their natural state. For example, the refining of rice using new milling techniques in twentieth-century Asia caused a scourge of *beriberi*, a thiamine-deficiency disease, which resulted in millions of deaths. Another such example is the substitution of bottle-feeding for breast-feeding among poor families in developing countries. This practice has been responsible for a great deal of malnutrition, diarrhea, and death.

Perhaps the most significant trend has been the gradual change from a variety of carbohydrates to a dependence on grains, especially hybridized wheat. We now know that heavy consumption of grains and beans has contributed to diabetes, cardiovascular disease, obesity, and many other serious illnesses. These foods are particularly high in lectins that react, in varying degrees, to all blood types.

Another trend that has had negative consequences for our health is the refining of sugar and the hydrogenization of fat. The meat our ancestors ate was very lean and rangy. Today's ranchers wouldn't think of trying to sell that meat. The marbled, fatty flavor of beef has become the standard for Western taste buds. The kind of meat that allowed humanity to thrive—lean, organic, and free of chemicals, pesticides, and hormones—was a far cry from a fatty T-bone steak or double cheeseburger.

Beyond the Balanced Diet

FOR SOME TIME NOW, physicians and nutritionists have equated a healthy diet with a balanced diet. *Balance* was defined as eating the recommended daily requirements deemed necessary for basic wellness. The only variations considered in the RDAs (Recommended Daily Allowances) published by the USDA are for age and sex (with the sole exception of pregnant and lactating women). In other words, our nutritional experts have stated that the vast array of other human differences does not affect this equation.

This is a classic example of reductionism: Take the entire population and reduce it down to the measurable commonalities—age and sex—and build your premise from those commonalities. This model works pretty well in conditions of starvation, or in emergencies and natural disasters. The question is, why have we built our entire nutritional foundation on a model that is meant for the basest level of subsistence? Reductionist nutritional advice is nothing more than nutrition for the lowest common denominator.

Polymorphism, on the other hand, is the true model for human nutrition. We are polymorphic beings whose individual differences are recorded in each cell of our bodies.

But conventional diet theory has a fundamental flaw. It is primarily devoted to identifying the effects of diet upon disease. It seeks to discover a set of statistically common problems, based on relatively small clinical trials, that may be related to diet, and to treat those conditions in a simple and logical manner. This approach is supported by the greater body of basic scientific knowledge, which is heavily influenced by societal norms, including big business. Corporate food and drug conglomerates make up the major funding sources for nutritional studies.

When *Eat Right 4 Your Type* was first published, I was often stunned when reviewers dismissed the theory out of hand by stating that there was no scientific research to support my claims. How could they say that when there are literally hundreds of articles published in scientific journals that support a blood type connection to diet and disease? It seemed to me that the so-called food authorities were so invested in promoting certain nutritional standards that they literally could not afford to accept a premise that did not fit into their modus operandi.

Conventional nutritional science is behind the curve. Blood type science is no longer relegated to a dusty cubicle, nor are naturopathic doctors like myself considered outside the mainstream. Indeed, many of the strongest supporters of my efforts are medical doctors who recommend the Blood Type Diet to their patients because it works. And the public itself is racing ahead of the standard theories of nutrition—which they often find too nonspecific to make a real difference.

The USDA Food Pyramid and the older "Four Basic Food Group" theory represent a uniform approach to human nutrition. However, since they are based on a concept of disease treatment, their recommendations revolve around the prevention of deficiency diseases. Vitamin C, an important component of our immune system, is only recommended in amounts (64mg/day) sufficient to prevent scurvy, a deficiency disorder. Yet it is known that in instances of infection and in many other disease states, our need for vitamin C can rise twentyfold. The prevention of deficiency diseases has little to do with functional need in our society, so the recommendations are for the most part useless in more specific treatment.

These dietary recommendations do have their value, however. They attempt to rectify malnutrition, which is a major worldwide dietary problem. They now promote the use of high-fiber whole foods rather than processed foods, which for the average Westerner is a major step forward. Unfortunately, conventional dietary recommendations are just that—conventional. What if you're not suffering from malnutrition and have already begun using whole foods? Unlike Hippocrates, who counseled, "Let your food be your medicine and let your medicine be your food," our modern nutritional principles are based on a separation of food and medicine. The Blood Type Diet allows us to restore the interrelationship of the two. We have accomplished this by studying a diverse collection of factors, some of which would seem to be unrelated to the specific science: anthropology, genetics, immunological responses, disease, and so on.

When you choose your diet based on a comprehensive understanding of all these factors, you will find—perhaps to your amazement—that you have not *chosen* a diet at all. The truth is, the correct diet has already been chosen for you by your blood type.

Blood Type and the USDA Food Pyramid

For certain blood types, the Food Pyramid recommendations make a fair amount of sense. Fundamentally, however, the pyramid is based on the reductionistic model we discussed earlier, meaning that it doesn't take into consideration dietary variations. For example, Type Os should *not* follow the basic pyramid recommendation of six to eleven servings of grain-based foods each day. And only Type B will benefit by eating the recommended amount of dairy foods. The Food Pyramid is probably closest to the needs of Type A. However, even foods within categories—which are not distinguished from one another in this model—can have a huge impact. For example, while Type Bs thrive on regular portions of meat, chicken can cause havoc in their digestive and immune systems.

My best advice is that you shouldn't try to fit a square peg into a round hole. Create your own Food Pyramid based on the foods that are listed on your blood type charts. All types should eat the recommended three to five servings of fruits and vegetables daily, but there is a wide divergence of choices in the level above, with two to three servings of dairy products recommended as well as two to three servings of meat, poultry, fish, beans, eggs, and nuts. For some blood types, such recommendations can be a very poor choice, indeed! The top of the pyramid, in which fats, oils, and sweets are located, recommends using these items sparingly, ignoring the fact that for many people 40 percent or more of their diets are from this section. The Food Pyramid was created to help Americans understand what a healthy diet entails. As with many other things, we've grown more sophisticated in our assessments of such recommendations. They seem well-meaning but inadequate. The pyramid really was created to provide minimal nutritional standards that would avoid malnutrition. As with many guidelines, the data are far too broad to really shed light on individual needs.

The Difference That Food Makes

NUTRITION IS NOT an abstract science. Nutrition studies the relationship of the food we eat to the way our bodies function—and what could be more relevant than that? Before you can fully understand your Blood Type Diet, you need to know the basic essentials of nutrition. Nutrition concerns the intake of food and the body's digestive processes: metabolism, the liberation of energy, and the elimination of wastes. Nutrients are substances that are necessary for maintaining the normal functioning of our bodies. The foods we consume must contain adequate amounts of about forty-five to fifty highly important substances, as well as water and oxygen. From these our bodies manufacture the substances necessary for life. These essential nutrients include carbohydrates, lipids (fats), proteins, vitamins and minerals, oxygen, and water.

The conversion of food to energy is expressed as the calorie, a unit of heat. The metabolism of basic nutrients produces calories at varying rates. One gram of protein will yield four calories. One gram of carbohydrate will also yield four calories. One gram of fat will yield nine calories.

Nutrients can generally be divided into five categories. They are: proteins, carbohydrates, fiber, fats, and vitamins and minerals. Before we focus on individual blood type requirements, let's briefly look at the functions that these nutrients perform.

Proteins

Every cell in the human body contains protein, and dietary protein is necessary to replenish the supply. Protein is essential for the growth and repair of tissues. Proteins are constructed from compounds called *amino acids*. Thirteen of the twenty-two amino acids can be produced in our bodies. But the other nine need to be derived from food. Animal foods are composed of complete proteins, meaning that they supply all of these essential amino acids in the proper proportions necessary to maintain health. Vegetable proteins are incomplete. They need to be combined in particular ways to get the proper complement of amino acids. It is the protein portion of certain foods, such as legumes and seafood, that contain blood type agglutinating lectins, which is why there is such a variation in which protein sources are best for your type.

We don't eat protein in a pure state. The sources of protein in our food supply come bound with other nutrients. A piece of meat might be 20 percent fat. When you evaluate how much protein you're eating, you need to subtract the fat and other elements that have been added.

Carbohydrates

Carbohydrates have always been the most abundant food source. In the marketplace, they have also always been the least expensive of foods. Carbohydrates can be divided into two groups: simple and complex. Simple carbohydrates are the sugars, such as fructose, glucose, and galactose. Complex carbohydrates, which are comprised of chemical combinations of simple sugars and are converted into sugars in plants or in the human body, are supplied by the starches—grains, tubers, and some rhizomes and roots. Almost two-thirds of the food energy used by humans worldwide is derived from carbohydrates. The rest comes from fats and proteins.

Many carbohydrates contain fiber. Fiber is an essential element in the diet, even though it provides no nutrients. It consists of the indigestible materials in plant foods. Water-insoluble fibers, such as cellulose, are primarily found in whole wheat, wheat bran, and the skins of fruit and vegetables. Cellulose is converted by the bacteria in the colon into a fatty acid called *butyrate*, which is used as an energy source by the cells of the colon. Butyrate is also known to have a protective effect against colon cancer, and the conversion of cellulose to butyrate complements the scrubbing action of fiber, further enhancing its anticancer effects. Diets with sufficient fiber produce bulkier stools, which helps to avoid constipation and other disorders, such as diverticulosis. Fruits, vegetables, whole-grain breads, and products made from nuts and legumes are all sources of dietary fiber. Water-soluble fiber, found primarily in fruits, vegetables, beans, and oats, is believed to be a factor in reducing blood cholesterol. However, high-fiber foods tend to contain food lectins. A high-fiber diet is usually a high-lectin diet, so choose your sources of fiber carefully.

Fats

Fats, a concentrated food source of stored energy, are usually converted back into carbohydrates before being metabolized. Fats are widely distributed in nature, and can be found in meat, poultry, fish, dairy, oils, grains, nuts, seeds, vegetables, and fruits. They are involved in the formation of cell walls and the production of hormones. Fats also are crucial in the circulation and absorption of fat-soluble vitamins A, D, E, and K. The essential fatty acids, linoleic acid and alpha-linoleic acid, can only be supplied by fat in the diet. Without them, the cells of the body would be unable to remain intact, as these essential fatty acids allow them to transport and excrete substances without placing the inner contents of the cells at risk.

There is a lot of confusion about the role fat plays in our diets. First, remember that we must have dietary fat for survival. But fats have different effects on our bodies according to their chemical construction. We do not need to eat saturated fats, such as those found in animal products and certain oils. The essential fatty acids come from polyunsaturated fats, contained in foods such as fish, leafy green vegetables, nuts, and seeds. Foods that are high in monounsaturated fats, such as olive oil, are excellent choices, no matter what your diet, although they do not act as a replacement for the essential fatty acids. Another good source of fat is fish oil, which is polyunsaturated but constructed differently from other fats. It contains omega-3 fatty acids.

Vitamins & Minerals

Most foods contain several vitamins and minerals, both of which are essential to health. Vitamins are needed only in minute quantities, but are required for normal metabolism. There are currently thirteen known vitamins—nine water soluble and four fat soluble. Water-soluble vitamins include vitamin C and eight B vitamins. Fat-soluble vitamins include vitamins A, D, E, and K.

Minerals are inorganic dietary elements that are necessary, in varying amounts, for good health. Macrominerals—calcium, phosphorus, magnesium, sodium, potassium, and chloride—are needed in substantial amounts. Trace minerals—just as important, but needed in far smaller amounts—include iron, zinc, selenium, iodine, copper, fluoride, chromium, manganese, and molybdenum.

Your cellular use of vitamins and minerals is blood type specific. *Eat Right 4 Your Type* contains a lengthy discussion about where they fit into your diet. The food plans themselves take their importance into consideration, so for the most part you don't need supplements. As a rule of thumb, try to consume most of the vitamins and minerals in your diet in the form of food, so that they can be digested and metabolized the way nature intended.

This Is Where Blood Type Comes In

Although nutritional knowledge of foods is important, it is only a part of the blood type equation. To be sure, certain foods may be packed full of nutrients. But it is the way those foods are broken down in your particular system and the reaction of your specific blood type antigens that classify them as Highly Beneficial, Neutral, or Avoid in the Blood Type Diet. Your blood type is the safest guide to maneuvering through the complex world of nutrition.

The Blood Type Diet is not a new way to eat, although you may be introduced to certain foods that have not been common in the modern diet. The Blood Type Diet is really a very old way to eat—as old as life itself.

Eat Right for Your Type

The O, A, B, AB Road Maps

O N PAGES 79 THROUGH 111 YOU WILL FIND THE Blood Type Diet food charts for Type O, Type A, Type B, and Type AB. Each chart contains a list of Highly Beneficial, Neutral, and Avoid foods appropriate for each blood type. You will also find recommendations about portion sizes as well as variations that typically are present for different ethnic groups.

The information in this chapter is designed to supplement the charts. It will help you refine your diet further and understand the basis for the blood type recommendations.

Meat & Poultry

When *Eat Right 4 Your Type* was first published, there was quite a lot of publicity about the recommendation of meat as an important source of protein for Type Os and, to a lesser extent, for Type Bs. People wondered how meat, normally high in saturated fat and cholesterol, could be recommended for anyone. It's true that most of the meat consumed today is too fatty and that it has been contaminated by the indiscriminate use of hormones and antibiotics. Let me stress that the Blood Type Diet recommends lean, organic meats, which are an entirely different dietary choice.

TYPE O. Type Os thrive on a diet high in animal protein. With the original blood type, Os have the perfect digestive systems for meat—stomachs with a high acid level that break food down quickly and metabolisms that distribute it for maximum utility. Type Os may also consume all poultry, but it is secondary as a protein source to red meat and doesn't have the same beneficial properties.

If You're a Type O Vegetarian

Type Os who have been eating a meat-free diet until now may have trouble at first properly digesting meat. In the beginning, eat small portions of meat several times a week, and chew them thoroughly to aid digestion. If red meat is a problem for you, you might also try supplementing your diet with a little known ayurvedic herb, *Coleus forskolii*. *Coleus* has been shown to enhance energy levels in Type Os. In many respects, its effects on cellular storage are similar to the effects of red meat. *Coleus* may be a solution for Type Os who have a philosophical problem with eating red meat. You might utilize this herb in combination with fish and poultry.

TYPE A. While meat is used as fuel for Type Os, it is poorly absorbed and purified by Type As, who thrive on a diet of vegetable protein. Soy protein should provide the bulk of "meat" in the Type A diet. Seafood and tofu can replace meat. Meat is poorly digested, increases digestive toxins in the Type A system, and is stored not as muscle-building protein, but as fat. Occasional lean, organic chicken is acceptable, but it should be included as in the Asian style of cooking—almost as a condiment more than as a main course.

T Y P E   B . Type Bs do quite well on a variety of meats. Interestingly, because of the ancestral history of Type Bs, they are able to adapt more easily to dietary circumstances of either low or high protein. There also appears to be a direct connection between stress, autoimmune disorders, and the kind of protein sources Bs use. They do best on other forms of red meat—lamb, mutton, venison, and rabbit—as opposed to the more ubiquitous beef.

One important point: Type Bs must avoid chicken. In a society focused on chicken as a major food source, giving it up is one of the most difficult adjustments Type Bs are asked to make. But it's a crucial health factor. Chicken contains a Type B agglutinating lectin in its muscle tissue, particularly in the breast meat. This lectin disturbs your system and can potentially lead to strokes and autoimmune disorders. If you tend to eat chicken often, I suggest that you begin to substitute turkey.

T Y P E   A B . Type ABs are unique in their relationship to meat because their blood type contains elements of both Type A and Type B. Like Type As, Type Bs are encouraged to seek protein from seafood and tofu. And, like Type Bs, their systems can also accommodate alternative red meats, such as lamb, mutton, venison, and rabbit. Meat should be eaten in small portions to make it more digestible, since Type Bs don't produce enough stomach acid to effectively utilize and digest excessive animal protein.

Fish

The second most potent source of animal protein available, fish also contains the valuable omega-3 fatty acids. Entire cultures have survived on diets of fish. Civilizations grew along the shores of the sea and the banks of rivers. The oceans, seas, lakes, rivers, and streams often provided an incredible bounty. No wonder people thought there were gods in the water. What other explanation could there have been?

TYPE O. Type O has a lengthy seafood menu from which to choose. Seafood is the second most concentrated animal protein, and is best suited to Type Os of Asian and Eurasian descent, though other Type Os can choose from a wide variety of richly oiled cold-water fish. Fish oils are of particular importance to Type Os because certain blood-clotting factors that evolved as humans adapted to environmental changes were missing from the blood of early Type Os. For this reason, Type Os often have "thin" blood, resistant to clotting. Although fish oils tend to have a blood-thinning effect, this is not an issue for Type Os. I suspect that is because the way Type O genes influence blood thickness—through clotting factors—is inherently different from the way in which fish oils influence blood viscosity—through the adhesion of platelets. Fish oils can also be very effective in the treatment of inflammatory bowel disease, such as colitis or Crohn's disease, to which Type Os are susceptible. Seafood is also an excellent source of iodine, which regulates thyroid function. Type Os typically suffer from hypothyroidism, a condition in which an insufficient amount of thyroid hormone is produced. Seafood should become a regular component of the healthy Type O diet.

TYPE A. Type As can eat fish up to three or four times a week to complement vegetable protein. Avoid the delicate white fish, such as halibut, hake, sole, and flounder; they contain a lectin that can irritate the Type A digestive tract. Type A women with a family history of breast cancer should consider introducing the edible snail *Helix pomatia* (escargot) into their diets. It helps fight cancer in the following way: In a precancerous condition, the body's cells manufacture a protein that allows the cancer to spread. The snail lectin attaches to those cells and essentially

Try "Peter's Snails" in the recipe section (page 144). This old family recipe is easy to make and delicious.

takes away their internal passport, blocking their ability to spread. Fish oils are believed to be a factor in reducing heart disease, which makes them important for Type As.

TYPE B. Type Bs thrive on fish. Deep ocean fish rich in oils, like cod, are excellent for Type Bs, as are white fish, such as halibut, flounder, and sole. Shellfish should be assiduously avoided by all Type Bs, as they contain lectins disruptive to the Type B system. This prohibition includes lobster, shrimp, crabs, and clams. Many of the original Type Bs were ancient Hebrew tribes whose laws forbade the consumption of shellfish. Perhaps this dietary law was an implicit acknowledgment of the fact that shellfish was poorly digested by Type Bs. Since the publication of *Eat Right 4 Your Type*, we have discovered that salmon roe—eggs—may also contain a lectin that agglutinates Type B cells. Until more information is available, I suggest that you limit your intake of salmon.

TYPE AB. Type ABs also have a vast variety of beneficial fish and seafood, but like Type As, they should avoid the white fish halibut, hake, sole, and flounder, and like Type Bs, all shellfish. Type AB women who have a family history of breast cancer should consider including the edible snail *Helix pomatia* in their diets. Type ABs also share with Type Bs the caution about salmon.

Dairy & Eggs

All dairy foods originate from milk. The composition of whole cow's milk is approximately 4.9 percent carbohydrate, 3.5 percent fat, 3.5 percent protein, and 87 percent water. The equation varies from species to species of lactating mammals. Human milk is higher in fat, whereas goat's milk is lower in fat. Milk contains important amounts of most nutrients, but it is very low in iron, vitamin C, and niacin. Calcium and phosphorus levels in milk are very high. Vitamin A levels are high in whole milk, but in the production of skim milk this fat-soluble vitamin is removed. Milk contains all of the essential amino acids that qualify it as a complete-protein food.

Unfortunately, cow's milk is heavily adulterated with antibiotics, to such an extent that a measurable amount of antibiotic can be detected in the tissue of humans who drink milk. Recent information about the use of growth hormone in commercial milk production is worrisome. Several studies link growth hormones to the genesis of breast cancer in women and prostate cancer in men. Look for dairy products advertised as "free of growth hormone." Raw or unpasteurized milk is not recommended because it carries a risk of bacterial contamination.

Dairy products and eggs have been prized by mankind as a valuable source of protein. For eons the egg has been a symbol of fertility and an object of pagan and religious worship. Although our modern nutritional analyses show that most dairy products are high in saturated fat and cholesterol, and that eggs are especially high in cholesterol, in moderation they are still integral dietary animal protein.

Butter is a substance that seems to go in and out of nutritional fashion. We all know that butter is a dense fat that contains a high level of cholesterol, but this is only part of the picture. Butter is also a rich source of small-chain fatty acids, principally one called *butyric acid*, which has been shown to have beneficial effects on the colon and digestive tract. In many parts of the world, such as India and Pakistan, a form of clarified butter, called *ghee*, is freely used. Remarkably, the use of ghee has not been shown to produce higher levels of blood cholesterol in these societies. Also, since any remaining proteins are removed in processing, ghee is a pure fat, with no lectin activity.

TYPE O. Type Os may eat small amounts of dairy and some eggs each week, but they are a poor source of protein for this blood type. Instead, Type Os should take a daily calcium supplement, especially women, since dairy foods usually provide the best source of absorbable calcium. Type Os' systems are ill-designed for the consumption of cheese, although they may eat eggs three to four times a week.

Type Os of African ancestry should completely eliminate eggs and dairy from their diet, because these foods are even harder for them to digest than for other Type Os. Lactose intolerance in the majority of people of African ancestry is logical because dairy wasn't eaten by their ancestors.

A word here about the difference between food allergies and food intolerances. Food *allergies* are not digestive problems. They are immune-system reactions to certain foods. Your immune system literally creates an antibody that fights a particular food's intrusion into your system. Food *intolerances* are digestive reactions, and can occur for many reasons. Poor-quality food, additives, psychological associations, cultural conditioning, or a particular quirk in someone's system can be the cause of an adverse reaction.

TYPE A. Most dairy products are not favorable for Type As, as this blood type creates antibodies to the primary sugar in whole milk, D-galactose. As you may recall, D-galactose is the essential sugar that forms the Type B antigen. The Type A immune system creates antibodies to reject B-like antigens, which would include whole-milk products. This perhaps explains why Type As tend to secrete a lot of mucus when they eat diary foods. If you suffer from a sinus condition or asthma, eliminate dairy altogether.

Calcium Alert

Because dairy foods are not generally favorable to Type Os, Type Os need to supplement their calcium intake, especially because they have a tendency to develop inflammatory joint pain and arthritis. I recommend 600 to 1,100 milligrams of elemental calcium every day for both adults and children.

Type As can tolerate small amounts of fermented dairy products like yogurt, kefir, and nonfat sour cream. Goat's milk is an excellent substitute for cow's milk. And, of course, soy milk and soy cheeses are excellent replacements for the Type A system.

Type As should limit egg consumption to the occasional organically grown egg. They are not an optimum Type A protein source.

TYPE B. Type B is the only blood type that can fully enjoy a variety of dairy products. The primary sugar in whole milk, D-galactose, is the primary sugar in the Type B antigen. The domestication of animals and dairy foods rose to prominence in the human diet as Type Bs reached the height of their development. However, even Type Bs should avoid eating sharp, hard cheeses, as they are not easily digestible. Eggs, by the way, do *not* contain the lectin found in the muscle tissue of chicken that makes it a food to avoid for Type Bs.

TYPE AB. Type ABs are in the betwixt and between world with regard to dairy products and eggs. They can enjoy some dairy products like a Type B, but the Type A–approved dairy foods, such as yogurt, kefir, and nonfat sour cream, are more easily digested. What Type AB should watch out for is excessive mucus production. Signs of respiratory problems, sinus attacks, or ear infections probably indicate a need to curtail consumption of dairy products.

Eggs are a very good source of protein for Type ABs. However, protein intake can be maximized by using two egg whites for every egg yolk.

Oils & Fats

In our haste to become a low-cholesterol society, many vegetable oils of low nutritional value are hawked to the unwitting consumer as being low in cholesterol. This may be true, but it is really beside the point. Plants and vegetables do not manufacture cholesterol, which is found only in animal products. Indeed, your non-cholesterol–containing vegetable oil may have little to recommend it. Tropical oils, such as coconut oil, are high in saturated fat.

Most oils sold today, including safflower and canola, are polyunsaturated, which makes them an improvement over tropical oils and animal fats such as lard. However, there is some concern that overconsumption of polyunsaturated fats may be linked to certain types of cancer, especially if you subject them to high temperatures in cooking. If you must heat your oils, use sesame, walnut, or peanut oils, which can tolerate high temperatures better. But the best alternative is to use olive oil in cooking as much as possible. As a monounsaturated fat, it actually has a beneficial effect on the heart and arteries.

Many people believe that margarine is a healthy alternative to butter. However, naturopathic doctors have known for some time that this is not true, and mainstream science is now acknowledging that fact. Margarine is produced by chemically altering a vegetable oil so that it becomes solid at room temperature. This is done by hydrogenating the oil, a process by which hydrogen is chemically added to oil, providing a higher melting point and thus solidifying it. The process causes the molecular configuration of the oil to change, producing trans–fatty acids (TFAs), which are potentially toxic, carcinogenic forms of fat. Add to this the liberal use of yellow coloring and chemical flavorings to pro-

---

Better Butter for Os and Bs

Mix together ½ pound of unsalted butter, ¼ cup of flaxseed or safflower oil, depending on your type, and 3 tablespoons of lecithin granules. Open a 400 i.u. vitamin E capsule with a pin and squeeze the contents into the mixture. Whip until stiffened. Better Butter should be refrigerated and will last about a week.

duce a butterlike look and feel, and you end up with a terrible alternative to butter. You'll find margarine listed occasionally in the recipe section. If you use it, do so sparingly.

I also recommend that all blood types use a tablespoon or two each day of flaxseed oil (linseed) or olive oil to aid in elimination.

TYPE O. Type Os can use oils as an important source of nutrition. They are best able to use flaxseed or olive oil. These oils have positive effects on the heart and arteries, and may help to lower cholesterol levels.

TYPE A. Type As need very little fat in their diet to function well. A tablespoon of olive or flaxseed oil each day has beneficial effects on elimination, cholesterol, and the heart. Type As should avoid corn and safflower oils; lectins in these oils cause digestive problems.

TYPE B. Since Type Bs respond very well to olive oil, they should use at least a tablespoon each day. Sesame, corn, and sunflower oils are antagonistic to the Type B digestive tract. Flaxseed oil is neutral for Type Bs. Clarified butter, or ghee, may be used in limited amounts by Type Bs.

TYPE AB. Type ABs do best with olive oil as opposed to other vegetable oils, hydrogenated oils, or animal fats. Ghee may be used in limited amounts.

Nuts & Seeds

Nuts and seeds have been as basic to humankind as they've been to the animals and birds of the Earth. However, there are very few nuts and seeds that are considered beneficial to *all* of the blood types. Many of them contain lectins. While they can be an important source of minerals and protein, especially the sulfur-containing amino acids, which help the body to detoxify, nuts and seeds can become rancid quite rapidly when they are exposed to air. Always keep nuts in closed containers. Do not grind your own nut butters at health food stores. This can result in dangerous levels of aflatoxin, a fungal poison. All prepared nut butters are already tested for aflatoxin.

Avoid processed nuts or nuts with high salt concentrations. People with gall bladder problems, appendicitis, or diverticulitis should avoid whole nuts and use nut butters instead.

TYPE O. Although Type Os can find a rich source of supplemental vegetable proteins from some varieties of nuts and seeds, they don't usually need them in their diet. Type Os trying to lose weight should completely avoid nuts, which are high in fat and calories. Only pumpkin seeds (rich in zinc) and walnuts are considered highly beneficial for Type Os. Be advised that nuts may exacerbate digestive problems for Type Os with problem colons.

TYPE A. There are many nuts and seeds that can provide a rich protein component to the Type A diet. Pumpkin and sunflower seeds, as well as almonds and walnuts, are excellent for Type As. Peanuts are highly beneficial for Type As because they contain a cancer-fighting lectin. Also it is beneficial to eat the papery outer skin of the peanut (not the shells!). Remember, however, that commercially grown peanuts tend to contain higher traces of toxins from the pesticides sprayed on them as they grow. Try to find organically grown peanuts. Those who have gall bladder problems should limit themselves to small amounts of nut butter rather than whole nuts.

TYPE B. Type Bs don't really do that well with nuts and seeds. Peanuts, sesame seeds, and sunflower seeds, among others, contain lectins that interfere with Type B insulin production. Although it may be difficult for many Type Bs of Asian and Middle Eastern origins to give up sesame seeds and other sesame-based products, blood type speaks more definitively in this instance than does culture. Nuts and seeds have the potential to make Type Bs quite ill.

TYPE AB. Nuts and seeds present a mixed opportunity for Type AB. Although they are a good source of supplementary protein, all seeds contain the insulin-inhibiting lectins that make them ill-advised for Type Bs. On the other hand, like Type As, Type ABs have a highly beneficial response to peanuts, which are powerful Type AB immune boosters. Type ABs have a propensity toward gall bladder problems, so nut butters in limited amounts are preferable to whole nuts.

Beans & Legumes

Although beans and legumes are central to cultures worldwide, each of the blood types has its own unique reactions. Beans and legumes are a common source of dietary lectins and are quite blood type specific. Most of the negative reactions concern an effect on insulin production.

TYPE O. Beans aren't well utilized by Type Os, although those of Asian ancestry react a little better because of acculturation. But in general, beans inhibit the metabolism of other, more important nutrients, such as those found in meat. Beans also tend to make muscle tissue slightly less acidic, and Type Os perform best when their muscle tissues are more acidic. This isn't to be confused with the acid/alkaline reaction that occurs in your stomach. In that instance, the few highly beneficial beans are exceptions. They actually strengthen the digestive tract and promote healing of ulcerations—a Type O problem because of high levels of stomach acid. Eat beans in moderation or as an occasional side dish.

TYPE A. Type As thrive on beans and legumes, as they provide a well-assimilated vegetable protein. Use caution in your selection, since not all beans and legumes are good for the Type A system. Some, such as the garbanzo, kidney, lima, and navy, contain a lectin that can slow insulin production. Slowed insulin production is a factor in both obesity and diabetes.

TYPE B. Kidney, lima, navy, and soy are the only beans that Type Bs should eat. Many beans and legumes contain lectins that interfere with the production of insulin. This is a contributing factor to the Type B tendency toward hypoglycemia. Type Bs of Asian ancestry tolerate beans and legumes somewhat better because of cultural acclimation. Still, limit the selection of such foods only to those that are highly beneficial, and eat sparingly of them.

TYPE AB. Type ABs exist in a realm of their own once again. Beans and legumes are a mixed bag of benefits and cautions. Lentil beans are an important cancer-fighting food for Type AB, but they're not recommended for Type B. Kidney and lima beans, known to slow insulin production in Type As, have the same effect on Type AB.

Soy

Soybeans and soy products are such an important blood type–specific dietary factor that they deserve a category of their own. The cultivation of soybeans in China predates recorded history and spread from there to other countries in eastern Asia before the modern period. So essential was the soy bean to Chinese civilization that it was considered one of the five sacred grains (the others being rice, barley, wheat, and millet). In the late nineteenth century the soybean plant attracted the attention of the U.S. Department of Agriculture, which began introducing improved soybean varieties through selective breeding. This program led to the introduction of varieties that differed markedly from the original Asian plants. The rapid increase in production in a period of little more than thirty years is one of the most striking developments in American agricultural history.

Soybeans can be an important human food because they are unusually rich in complete proteins. For Blood Type A, soy is as valuable—and should be as cherished—as any of the animal proteins previously listed. Soy is a miracle bean—potent with vital protein and capable of being transformed into a vast multitude of other foods.

Soybeans can be eaten roasted, dried, crushed, or boiled. Soy can be turned into oil, milk, and flour, or altered to become tofu, tempeh, okara, miso, cheese, or textured vegetable protein. Just recently, scientists have announced that soy can be used as an alternative fuel source, and even transformed into a textile. For our purposes, however, we will concentrate on soy as food. Soy is a staple as intrinsic to the world food supply as was maize to the ancient Inca, Maya, and Aztec civilizations.

TYPE O. Soy is a neutral food for Type Os, and therefore is not an ideal protein choice. Other sources of high-quality protein, such as meat and fish, are preferable.

TYPE A. Type As are encouraged to use soy products in place of animal protein. Type A systems respond very favorably to soy, which is also a great protector against cancer. Soy's lectins agglutinate and sweep A-like mutated cells from the system, and soy is easily assimilated digestively. Type As thrive on vegetable protein, and soy provides an extremely nutritious source.

TYPE B. Type Bs are advised to limit tofu and other soy products because they essentially have no immune payoff. The cancer protection from soy is Type A specific. Type Bs really need meat, dairy, and fish as their primary protein sources to enjoy optimum health. However, many Asian societies contain high numbers of Type Bs in their populations. Soy is an elemental part of Asian cuisine, so many Type Bs regularly eat soy. I recommend that you moderate your intake of soy products and substitute small amounts of meat and fish.

TYPE AB. Type ABs tolerate soy exceptionally well. They derive from soy the same cancer-fighting benefits as Type A. Soy is also an excellent choice for Type ABs who want to lose weight.

Grains

Grains provide abut 70 percent of the food energy that we consume. The most commonly cultivated and consumed are rice,
wheat, and corn, closely followed by millet, sorghum, oats, and
barley. Other major energy sources are the tuber and root crops,
such as potatoes, beets, and carrots. The fat content of grain
products is usually low, unless the germ is retained in the processing. Whole-grain products contribute significant quantities of
fiber as well as trace vitamins and minerals such as pantothenic
acid, vitamin E, zinc, copper, manganese, and molybdenum.
However, some grains are also a rich source of a class of lectins
called *glutens,* and these can be quite blood type specific.

In our society, corn and wheat products are ubiquitous. Think
about it. How many labels have you read that did not contain the
words "corn sweetener"? Even rye bread is only 30 percent rye
and 70 percent wheat. This poses distinct blood type–related
problems.

How do you get around it? Health-food stores can be a bo-
nanza here. Also refer to the mail-order resources listed in the ap-
pendix. In recent years, many ancient grains, largely forgotten,
have been rediscovered and are now being produced. Examples
are amaranth, a grain from Mexico, and spelt, a variation of wheat
that seems to be free of the problems found in whole wheat.
Spelt flour makes a hearty, chewy bread that is quite flavorful.
You may have noticed that several popular breakfast cereals are
currently being made from amaranth.

All blood types should take advantage of sprouted-wheat
breads. Essene and Ezekiel bread, also known as "Bible breads,"
are sprouted-seed breads that are wonderful, live foods with
many of their beneficial enzymes still intact. The gluten lectin,
found principally in the seed coat, is destroyed by the sprouting
process. These breads can usually be found in the freezer section
of your health-food store because they spoil rapidly. Sprouted
breads are somewhat sweet tasting, as the sprouting process also

releases sugars. They are also moist and chewy. Beware of commercially produced sprouted-wheat breads, as they usually are largely whole wheat, with only a small amount of sprouted wheat. Always read the ingredients on the label.

Many people worry about the yeast content of breads causing problems, especially if they suffer from irritable bowel syndrome or have read any of the "yeast connection" theories. Frankly, I have not seen this as a problem. I suspect that what many people believe to be a reaction to the yeast in bread is actually a reaction between the gluten lectins and the blood type chemicals in their digestive tracts.

TYPE O. Wheat products aren't tolerated by Type Os at all. Eliminate wheat from the Type O diet. Wheat contains lectins that react with the Type O digestive tract and blood, and interfere with the proper absorption of beneficial foods. Wheat also causes weight gain for Type Os because glutens in wheat germ interfere with metabolic processes. Slowed metabolism causes food to convert to energy sluggishly. As a result, it stores itself as fat. There are no highly beneficial cereals recommended for Type O. When eating pasta, choose pastas made of buckwheat, Jerusalem artichoke, rice flour, or quinoa. Although oat products are on the Type O Avoid list, you may eat them occasionally if you're not suffering from digestive problems or trying to lose weight.

Watch Out for Wheat!

Wheat is the most ubiquitous ingredient in all packaged goods, from sauces to noodles. You'll even find wheat hiding out in corn cereals, rye bread, and rice preparations. Sauces and thickeners are often wheat based. Read the labels.

TYPE A. Cereals and grains can be eaten one or more times every day by Type As. Whole grains should be chosen over more processed cereals. Type As with mucus conditions caused by asthma, or frequent sinus infections, should limit wheat consumption, as wheat causes increased mucus production. Type As must also balance the acid-forming wheat with alkaline foods (see fruits). Type As perform best when their tissues are slightly alkaline, in direct contrast to Type Os: While the inner kernel of wheat grain is alkaline in Type Os, it becomes acidic in Type As.

TYPE B. Balance is the key for Type B, who should eat a variety of cereals. Rice and oats are excellent choices. Wheat contains a lectin that attaches to the insulin receptors and interferes with insulin efficiency, which causes weight gain. Type Bs should also avoid rye, which contains a lectin that settles in the vascular system and can cause blood disorders and potential strokes. Corn and buckwheat are major culprits in Type B weight gain. More than any other food for Type B, they contribute to a sluggish metabolism, insulin irregularity, fluid retention, and fatigue. Try spelt, which is highly beneficial for Type B.

TYPE AB. Type ABs do best when their tissues are slightly alkaline, so like Type A, they should limit their wheat consumption, especially if they need to lose weight or have a mucus condition. They also share Type B's sensitivity to the lectins in buckwheat and corn. Type ABs are advised to eat a diet that includes rice, oats and rye, although it is permissible to eat wheat products once or twice a week.

Vegetables

Most vegetables are good sources of vitamins, minerals, and fiber. Certain vegetables, such as potatoes and corn, contribute appreciable quantities of starch to the diet. Large amounts of calcium and iron can be found in some vegetables, particularly beans, peas, and broccoli. Vegetables also supply sodium chloride, cobalt, copper, magnesium, manganese, phosphorus, and potassium. Carotenes, the precursor of vitamin A and vitamin C, are abundant in many vegetables. Vegetables also contain helpful amounts of fiber, and provide the roughage required to promote the proper movement of food through the intestines.

TYPE O. There are a tremendous number of vegetables available to Type Os, and they form a critical component of the Type O diet. However, several classes of vegetables create problems for Type Os. The Brassica family—cabbage, Brussels sprouts, cauliflower, and mustard greens—can affect thyroid function, which is already somewhat deficient in Type Os. Leafy green vegetables rich in vitamin K, like kale, collard greens, romaine lettuce, broccoli, and spinach, are very good for Type Os. Vitamin K helps blood clot, and Type Os lack several clotting factors. Alfalfa sprouts contain components that can aggravate Type O hypersensitivity problems by irritating the digestive tract. The molds in domestic and shiitake mushrooms as well as in fermented olives tend to trigger allergic reactions in Type Os. Nightshade vegetables, such as eggplant and potatoes, can cause arthritic conditions in Type Os, because their lectins deposit in the tissue surrounding the afflicted joints. Corn lectins affect the production of insulin, which can lead to obesity and diabetes. All Type Os should avoid corn, especially if they have a weight problem or a family history of diabetes. Tomatoes are heavily laced with powerful lectins called *panhemaglutinans*. Panhemaglutinans agglutinate all blood types. However, Type Os can occasionally eat tomatoes because they don't stimulate the production of antibodies, and they become neutral in the Type O digestive system.

TYPE A. Vegetables are a crucial part of the Type A diet and should be consumed raw or steamed to preserve the most nutrients. Peppers aggravate the Type A digestive system, as do the molds in fermented olives. The lectins in domestic potatoes, sweet potatoes, yams, and cabbage should also be avoided. Avoid tomatoes, that rare vegetable classified as a panhemaglutinan, which has a deleterious effect on the Type A system. Although corn is on the Type A neutral list, I suggest you avoid it if you have digestive problems or want to lose weight. Maitaki mushrooms are revered in Japan as a powerful tonic for the immune system. Recent studies show that they have anticancer properties, which make them highly beneficial for Type As. Yellow onions contain a bioflavinoid called *quercitin*, which is a powerful antioxidant. Broccoli is highly recommended for its antioxidant benefits. Other beneficial vegetables include carrots, collard greens, kale, pumpkin, and spinach. Garlic, a natural antibiotic and immune-system booster, is also good for the blood.

TYPE B. For the most part, Type Bs can claim the vegetable world as their kingdom, with a few caveats. Tomatoes must be eliminated from the Type B diet. The panhemaglutinans produce a strong reaction, usually in the form of irritation of the stomach lining. Corn contains lectins that upset Type B insulin production and metabolic functions. Olives should also be avoided because their molds can trigger allergic reactions. As Type Bs are particularly vulnerable to viruses and autoimmune disorders, they should eat plenty of leafy greens, which contain magnesium, an important antiviral agent. Magnesium is also helpful for Type B children suffering from eczema. Unlike the other blood types, Type Bs can enjoy potatoes, yams, and cabbage.

TYPE AB. Fresh vegetables are an important source of phytochemicals, the substances in foods that help prevent cancer and heart disease—diseases that afflict Type A and Type ABs more frequently because of their weaker immune systems. Nearly all of the vegetables that are good for Type A and Type B are good for Type ABs. The exception is tomatoes. Type ABs have so much blood type material that they can enjoy the nonspecific tomato lectin with no ill effect.

Fruits

As with vegetables, we have been blessed with a vast and delicious array of rich, nutritious, and beneficial fruits. Vegetables that are botanically fruits include avocado, squash, tomato, eggplant, olives, and nuts. Each of the blood types has a generous list of highly beneficial and neutral fruits, with only a few fruits that are specifically to be avoided.

Citrus fruits are a valuable source of vitamin C, and the yellow fruits, such as peaches, contain carotene. Figs are an excellent source of calcium, and dried fruits not only are a concentrated source of sugar but also contain an ample amount of iron. Grapes, plums, berries, apples, and pears, all contribute to the treasure available to humankind. And, like vegetables, fruits have a high fiber content.

TYPE O. Fruits not only are an important source of vitamins, minerals, and fiber, but they can be an excellent alternative to breads and pasta for Type Os. A piece of fruit will serve the Type O system far better than a slice of bread, and will promote weight loss, too. Plums, prunes, and figs are highly beneficial to Type Os. That's because most dark red, blue, and purple fruits tend to cause an alkaline reaction in the Type O digestive tract. The alkaline reaction helps reduce irritations of the stomach lining. However, not all alkaline fruits are good for Type O. Melons are alkaline, but they contain a lot of mold, to which Type Os have a proven sensitivity. Cantaloupe and honeydew, which have the highest mold counts of all, should be avoided. Oranges, tangerines, and strawberries should be avoided because of their high acid content. Grapefruit also has a high acid content, but it exhibits alkaline properties after consumption so it can be included in the Type O diet. Most berries are fine, but blackberries contain a lectin that aggravates Type O digestion. Coconuts and products containing coconut should be avoided by Type Os, who exhibit an extreme sensitivity to it. Check food labels to make sure no coconut oil is present.

TYPE A. Type As should eat fruit three times a day. They should try to emphasize the more alkaline fruits such as berries and plums, which can help to balance the acid forming in their muscle tissue because of the grains that Type As should be consuming. High mold counts in melons should warn Type As off, and cantaloupe and honeydew melons should be avoided altogether. Type As don't tolerate tropical fruits such as mango and papaya, which cause indigestion. Other high-potassium fruits that might substitute for bananas are apricots, figs, and certain melons. Pineapple, however, is an excellent digestive aid for Type As. Oranges are a stomach irritant for Type As, and should be avoided. Grapefruits and lemons are excellent for Type As. Grapefruit has a positive alkaline effect after digestion, and lemons aid digestion and clear mucus from the Type A system.

TYPE B. Type Bs tend to have very balanced digestive systems, so they can enjoy many of the fruits that are upsetting to other blood types. There are very few fruits that Type Bs are advised to abstain from: Persimmons, pomegranates, and prickly pears won't be sorely missed. Pineapple contains a digestive enzyme, called *bromelain*, that can help reduce water retention in Type Bs as they become accustomed to this diet.

Type Bs should try to eat at least two or three servings every day of the fruits on the Type B Highly Beneficial list to take advantage of their pro-B medicinal qualities.

TYPE AB. Type ABs inherit mostly Type A intolerances and preferences for certain fruits. Grapes, plums, and berries are more alkaline fruits that can help balance the acid formed in the tissues by the consumption of grain. Type AB should avoid tropical fruits such as bananas, mangoes, and guava. Pineapple, however, is an excellent digestive aid for Type AB. Oranges are a stomach irritant for Type AB and interfere with the absorption of important minerals. Lemons and grapefruit, on the other hand, are excellent for the Type AB digestive system. Grapefruit ex-

hibits alkaline tendencies after digestion, and lemons aid digestion and clear mucus from the system.

Juices & Fluids

The recommendations for fruit and vegetable juices mirror the
blood type recommendations regarding vegetables and fruits for
each type.

TYPE O. Vegetable juices are preferable to fruit juices for Type
Os because of their alkalinity. If a Type O does drink a fruit juice,
it should contain less sugar than apple juice or cider. Pineapple
juice, while quite sweet, contains the enzyme *bromelain,* which
can be particularly helpful in avoiding water retention and bloating. Black cherry is also a beneficial, high-alkaline juice for the
Type O system.

TYPE A. Each day should begin with a small glass of warm
water into which the juice of one-half lemon has been squeezed.
This will clear the mucus that has accumulated overnight in the
more sluggish Type A digestive tract and stimulate elimination.
Alkaline fruit juices should be consumed in preference to highly
sugared juices, which are more acid forming.

TYPE B. Most fruit and vegetable juices are perfectly all right
for Type B. There is a special beverage for Type Bs, which some
of my readers have dubbed "Membrosia." The recipe calls for 1
tablespoon of flaxseed oil, 1 tablespoon of high-quality lecithin
granules, and 6 to 8 ounces of a fruit juice of choice. Lecithin is
an enzyme found in animals and plants that contain metabolism-
and immune system–enhancing properties. Membrosia provides
high levels of choline, serine, and ethanolamine, all phospho-
lipids of great value to the Type B system. This beverage is actually tastier than one might imagine, as the lecithin emulsifies and
mixes with the oil, allowing it to blend with the juice.

TYPE AB. Begin each day with a small glass of warm water into which the juice of one-half lemon has been squeezed. This will help clear the sluggish Type AB digestive system of mucus and will also aid in elimination. A glass of diluted grapefruit or papaya juice should be enjoyed afterward. Stress high-alkaline fruit juices for the Type AB system: black cherry, cranberry, or grape.

Spices & Herbs

We often think of spices and herbs as being interchangeable, but they are really quite different. Spices are extracted from bark, flower buds, fruits, roots, and seeds. Herbs are green-leafed plants originally found in temperate zones and grown today in many home gardens. Spices and herbs contain surprising amounts of nutrients. Not only do they improve the taste of much of what we eat, but many herbs and spices contain powerful medicinal properties.

TYPE O. Spices can actually improve the Type O digestive and immune systems. Kelp-based seasonings are rich sources of iodine, key to regulating the thyroid gland. Iodized salt is another good source of iodine, but use it sparingly. The fucose in bladderwrack provides a molecule that blocks the bacteria that attack your stomach lining and cause ulcers. Kelp is also a highly effective metabolic regulator for Type Os, and is an important aid to weight loss. Parsley, like most green vegetables, helps blood to clot. Certain warming spices, such as curry and cayenne pepper, are soothing for Type Os. Vinegar irritates the Type O stomach, and Type Os may have an allergic reaction to black pepper. Sugar and honey won't harm Type Os, nor will chocolate, but they should all be limited to occasional use. Corn syrup and sweeteners should be avoided.

TYPE A. Spices are more than just flavor enhancers for Type As; they can provide powerful immune-boosting properties. Soy-

---

The Sweet-Tooth Factor

Many followers of the Blood Type Diet are elated to find sugar and chocolate on their Neutral lists. They're accustomed to being told to avoid these "bad" foods—a rule that seems punitive. Neither sugar nor chocolate contain blood type agglutinating lectins which are poisonous. However, just because they appear on the Neutral list doesn't mean they have no effect at all. Alone, sugar provides no nutritional benefit, nor does chocolate—although chocolate does contain caffeine. Other sweeteners, such as honey and syrup, are just as empty of nutrients as white sugar. Let common sense be your guide when it comes to a decision about eating "empty" foods.

---

based spices such as tamari, miso, and soy sauce are tremendously beneficial for Type A. To combat the high sodium inherent in these products, use lowered-sodium versions. Blackstrap molasses is an excellent source of iron, a mineral lacking in the Type A diet. Kelp is an excellent source of iodine and many other valuable minerals. Vinegar should be avoided, as the acid tends to irritate the Type A stomach lining. Sugar and chocolate are allowed on the Type A Diet, but in very small amounts. If possible, avoid white processed sugar altogether. Recent studies have shown that the immune system is sluggish for several hours after eating it. Hawthorn supplements are advised for Type As with a history of cardiovascular disease. This phytochemical increases the elasticity of the heart muscles and strengthens the heart. Immune-enhancing herbs, such as echinacea, can help ward off colds and flu.

TYPE B. Type Bs respond best to warming spices such as ginger, horseradish, curry, and cayenne pepper. Black and white pepper contain problem lectins for Type Bs. Sweet herbs tend to irritate the Type B stomach. Avoid barley-malt sweeteners, corn syrup, cornstarch, and cinnamon. Molasses, honey, and white and brown sugar react in a neutral way in the Type B system, so these sugars may be used in moderation. Type Bs can also tolerate small amounts of chocolate. Herbal preparations of Siberian ginseng and Ginko Baloba increase memory retention and concentration, sometimes a problem for Type Bs with nervous disorders.

TYPE AB. Instead of commercial table salt, Type ABs should use sea salt and kelp for their relatively low sodium content—a concern for Type AB. In addition to immensely positive heart and immune-system benefits, kelp is also helpful in weight control. Miso, derived from soy, is excellent for Type ABs, and makes a delicious broth or sauce. Type ABs need to avoid pepper and limit their consumption of vinegar. To dress vegetables or salads, Type ABs should use lemon juice with olive oil and garden herbs and use lots of garlic, which is a potent blood tonic and a natural antibiotic. Sugar and chocolate are allowed in very limited amounts.

Condiments

There is an enormous world of condiments, with many different definitions. Is mayonnaise a condiment? Is a pickle? Are relishes condiments? Of course, but there are so many. Mango chutney, lemon chutney, nut chutney, pickle relish, corn relish, tomato relish, onion relish, mustard relish. No wonder there's so much confusion. All involve concoctions of herbs, spices, vinegars, and marinades, some of which marry each other and some of which conflict. As with herbs and spices, condiments offer endless variations of hot, sour, sweet and bitter, pickled, peppered, preserved, and piquant. Many blood type–approved sauces and condiments that you can make yourself are included in the recipe section. Here we address basic commercial condiments.

TYPE O. There are no highly beneficial condiments for Type O. If you use mustard or salad dressing on your foods, limit their

---

Better Condiments for Your Blood

Try some of these creative alternatives to the standard toppings. Be sure to check the ingredients first.

Chili oil: A vegetable oil in which hot red chili peppers have been steeped to release heat and flavor. (Avoid for A.)

Chili powder: A combination of garlic, cumin, oregano, cloves, coriander, and dried chiles. (Avoid for A.)

Hoisin sauce: Sweet and spicy reddish brown sauce made from soybeans, garlic, chili peppers, and several spices. (Good substitute for standard soy sauces, which tend to have wheat in them.)

Miso: Soybean paste that now comes in powdered form to use as an easy addition to many recipes.

Tahini: A thick paste made from ground sesame seeds.

Tamari: Thicker than soy sauce, with a mellow flavor. Made from soybeans and excellent for basting meat or vegetable dishes.

---

consumption. Type Os can tolerate tomatoes, but ketchup contains ingredients such as vinegar and should be avoided. The same is true for mayonnaise. All pickled foods are indigestible for Type Os. They severely irritate the Type O stomach lining. Replace condiments with healthier seasonings such as olive oil, lemon juice, and garlic.

TYPE A. There are no beneficial condiments for Type A. Type As can have small quantities of jam and low-fat salad dressings. However, they should avoid pickles and pickled foods which have been linked to stomach cancer in people with low levels of stomach acid. Ketchup should be eliminated from the Type A Diet, as neither the tomato nor the vinegar is digestible.

TYPE B. They can handle almost all condiments with the exception of ketchup, which has dangerous lectins. However, intake should be limited to very small portions and occasional use.

TYPE AB. Type ABs should avoid all pickled condiments because of their susceptibility to stomach cancer.

Herbal Teas

Herbal teas provide most of the blood types with an enormous advantage. Concoctions of herbs have been used for eons to treat a host of illnesses, real and imagined. Today, they are widely available commercially and have been rightly restored to a place of honor in most homes.

TYPE O. Herbal teas can be used by Type Os to shore up their strength against natural weaknesses. The primary emphasis for Type Os is on soothing the digestive and immune systems. Licorice can soothe the stomach irritations that are common to Type Os. A licorice preparation called DGL can be found in health-food stores. It is safe to use because it does not contain the component in raw licorice that can raise blood pressure. Herbs such as peppermint, parsley, rose hips, and sarsaparilla all have a soothing effect. Alfalfa, aloe, burdock, and corn silk cause nonspecific immune stimulation of Type O, which can exacerbate immune diseases.

TYPE A. While the Type O system needs to be soothed, the Type A system needs to be revved up. The most outstanding health risk factors for Type As are related to their sluggish immune systems. Aloe, alfalfa, burdock, and echinacea are immune-system boosters. Green tea has a powerful antioxidant effect on the digestive tract, providing protection against cancer. Hawthorn is a cardiovascular tonic. Slippery elm, gentian, and ginger increase stomach-acid secretion. Chamomile and valerian root are excellent herbal relaxants for the Type A system.

TYPE B. There are a number of herbal teas that are highly beneficial for Type Bs. Ginger warms and peppermint soothes. Ginseng
has a positive effect on the nervous system. It has a stimulant effect, so be sure to drink it early in the day. Licorice is excellent
for Type Bs. It contains antiviral properties that work to reduce
the Type B susceptibility to autoimmune diseases. Also, many
Type Bs experience a drop in blood sugar levels after meals (hypoglycemia), and licorice helps regulate blood-sugar levels. I've
more recently discovered that licorice is a fairly powerful elixir for
those suffering from chronic fatigue syndrome. However, a caution
applies: Since it can raise blood pressure, never consume licorice
in supplements or licorice root without consulting your doctor.

TYPE AB. Herbal teas should be employed by Type ABs to rev
up the immune system and build protection against cardiovascular disease and cancer. Alfalfa, burdock, chamomile, and echinacea are immune-system boosters. Hawthorn and licorice are
recommended for cardiovascular health. Green tea has enormous
cancer-inhibiting properties and a positive effect on the immune
system. Dandelion, burdock root, and strawberry leaf teas aid the
absorption of iron and prevent anemia in Type AB.

Miscellaneous Beverages

Entire cultures gravitate to coffees, teas, wines, beers, and
liquors. Seltzers, tonics, sodas, and drinks of all kinds are an integral part of the lives of nations. Some of these beverages have
positive effects on certain blood types. Other beverages are best
avoided.

TYPE O. There seem to be few acceptable beverages for Type
Os. Seltzer and tea are pretty innocuous. Beer may be consumed
in moderation, but not if you're trying to lose weight. Small
amounts of wine are also allowed. Coffee increases already high
stomach-acid levels in Type O, so it is best if it's eliminated alto-

gether. Green tea is a good caffeinated alternative, although it has no special protective properties for Type Os.

TYPE A. Surprisingly, coffee is recommended for Type As because it increases the amount of stomach acid and has some of the same enzymes that are found in soy. Green tea should also be consumed regularly by Type As. Red wine is good for Type As because of its positive effect on the cardiovascular system. All other beverages should be avoided.

TYPE B. Type Bs thrive on herbal and green teas, water, and juice. Coffee, tea, and wine don't harm Type Bs, but they don't really help them, either. Since the goal of the Blood Type Diet is to maximize performance, the elimination of these unnecessary stimulants is a way to increase overall Type B performance.

TYPE AB. Coffee is recommended for Type ABs because it has a lot of the same enzymes found in soy. Green tea is also of benefit to Type ABs because of its powerful antioxidant capabilities. Red wine is good for Type ABs because of its cardiovascular benefits. Beer is of neutral benefit, but may be consumed in moderation.

These are the general guidelines concerning the foods that are right for your blood type. In the next chapter we'll get down to the practical matters that really make the diet work—shopping, preparing, and eating those foods—and perhaps most important—the best way to get started if you're new to the Blood Type Diet.

FIVE

Getting Started

From Mind-Set to
Market to Table

ONE OF THE MAIN REASONS PEOPLE GET TURNED OFF to diets is that the plans are so often cloaked in righteousness. There's a "my way or the highway" tone to them that leaves people jittery and afraid to diverge even the tiniest bit for fear of falling off their imaginary wagon.

I believe that the right dietary program is one that you grow into, not one that you jump into all in one day. It should feel comfortable and *right*, not like a straitjacket. That's one of the reasons I stay away from rigid calorie counts or complicated equations to determine the percentage of protein, fat, and carbohydrates in your diet. The portion sizes are likewise just broad recommendations. There will always be individual variations according to your height, weight, age, physical condition, and the availability of food. It is not my goal to strangle you with a diet. In order for you to truly eat the way nature intended, it has to feel natural. That can take time—and it certainly involves some flexibility.

If you have tried other diet plans—and most of you have— you're probably used to the feeling that something terrible will happen if you "go off" your diet. I can't tell you how many times people have contacted me in desperation because they have encountered a situation that is completely incompatible with the Blood Type Diet. I once had a woman call me, frantic, because she was going to her best friend's wedding and was worried about what would happen if she ate a piece of wedding cake. My answer was, "Well, I suppose you'll enjoy it." This is typical of the terrible anxiety people feel about food. Since anxiety is very bad for digestion, I don't encourage it. The fact is, if you're generally healthy, you can be flexible when the occasion demands it. Chances are, armies of lectins won't march in and destroy your fortress. I am a Type A who happens to love tofu. I've eaten it all my life. But about once every year or so I get a terrible craving for my wife Martha's stuffed cabbage with ground meat. And I don't feel guilty about the indulgence.

The point is, it's great if you are truly committed to the Blood Type Diet. But life is too short to worry about the pinch of cinnamon that's the eighth ingredient in your favorite recipe.

If You're New to the Blood Type Diet

YOU MAY BE eager to dive right into the diet that fits your blood type. But before you sweep your kitchen clean of any and all offending foods and go on a Highly Beneficial binge, take some time to learn what this diet is all about. The best way to introduce yourself to the Blood Type Diet is to follow these steps over a period of time:

1. READ *EAT RIGHT 4 YOUR TYPE* and don't just skip to the section about your own blood type. You can't understand the Type B factors unless you also understand the historical context—the evolutionary process that has contributed to the role blood type plays in every person's diet. And that's true for Types O, A, and AB, too. I know that people often follow diets that seem arbitrary to them. They're told, "Eat this, don't eat that,"

and they follow it to the letter. Maybe they get results; maybe they don't. But in the long run, nobody will abide by a method that doesn't live in their head and heart.

2. BEGIN BY ADDING FOODS TO YOUR DIET FROM THE HIGHLY BENEFICIAL LIST. Take a look at the foods that have a positive medicinal effect on your blood type. Start incorporating into your diet foods you are not already eating.

3. START EXERCISING FOR YOUR BLOOD TYPE. Exercise is a critical component of the Blood Type Diet. In *Eat Right 4 Your Type* you will find a full explanation of why different blood types do well on different regimens. Briefly, the recommendations are: Type O—intense physical exercise such as aerobics or jogging; Type A—calming, tension-relieving exercises such as yoga, walking, and Tai Chi; Type B—moderate activities such as hiking, cycling, and martial arts; and Type AB—the same calming exercises as Type A. It has been demonstrated that the combination of eating Highly Beneficial foods and doing the appropriate exercise makes a very big difference for beginners.

4. BEGIN TO ELIMINATE FOODS FROM YOUR AVOID LIST. Start looking for natural replacements for your Avoid foods. For example, a Type A who is accustomed to eating meat can start by replacing meat with fish and substituting chicken for beef or lamb. Your goal should be to gradually replace the Avoid items with Highly Beneficial and Neutral foods. When you read the descriptions of the interactions between certain foods and your blood type, you'll discover that some food lectins are particularly potent. Try to eliminate these first.

At the Market

YOU DON'T HAVE to be a food scientist or carry a gram counter or calculator when you go to the market. Simply focus on selecting

---

Blood Type–Priority Checklist

There are many reasons why people are not able to follow their Blood Type Diet completely. I am often asked, "If I could do just two or three things to make a difference in my diet, what would they be?" Here are some suggestions. They might also be helpful for those who are just getting started.

TYPE O: Begin eating small portions of lean red meat three to four times a week. Eliminate wheat.

TYPE A: Replace meat with vegetable protein, supplemented with fish. Add more beans and grains to your diet.

TYPE B: Start eating dairy foods several times a week and eliminate chicken.

TYPE AB: Make seafood, tofu, and small quantities of meat, such as lamb and turkey, your staples. Avoid chicken, corn, and most beans.

ALL BLOOD TYPES: Eat organic meat, poultry, vegetables, and fruit. If you can't afford to do that, start with meat and poultry, and wash your vegetables and fruit thoroughly. Exercise right for your blood type.

---

the freshest foods in their most natural state. And use your knowledge of basic nutritional principles. Here are a few tips:

Avoid heavily fatted meats. Free-range poultry and meats have been raised without the excessive use of antibiotics and other chemicals, and they're recommended for the Blood Type Diet. *Free range* means just that—that animals haven't been penned in. Once you try free-range meat or poultry, you'll see the difference. The flesh is leaner, the color and texture are richer, and there is very little fat. It's possible to raise red meats that have fat and cholesterol levels that are closer to those of the leaner poultry, but the meat may be less tender and flavorful by modern standards. The giant agribusinesses are still locked into the traditional notion that consumers want rich, high-fat meats. Our ancestors consumed rather lean game or domestic animals that grazed on alfalfa and other grasses. Today's meats are corn-fed, kept healthy with antibiotics, and prized for the tenderness of their meat and the marbling of their fat. Fortunately, some businesses are beginning to respond to the growing demand for lean, organic meat. If your market hasn't caught on to the trend, be sure to let the manager know.

Fresh fish is fairly simple to identify. Look at the eyes. If they are clear and reflective, the fish is probably fresh. Pull the gills out from back of the head. They should be bright red or dark pink. If the skin is slimy to the touch, or the fish has any kind of off odor or fishy smell, it is not fresh.

Try to avoid the canned-foods aisles. Commercially canned foods are subjected to high heat and pressure, and they lose a great deal of their vitamin content, especially the antioxidants, such as vitamin C. They do retain the vitamins that are not heat sensitive, such as vitamin A. Canned foods are usually lower in fiber and higher in salt. The salt is added to boost the flavor lost during production. Few of the natural enzymes remain; for the most part, they're destroyed by the canning process.

Other than fresh, frozen foods are your best bet, since freezing doesn't alter the nutritional content of the food very much. The quality and variety of frozen foods have improved greatly in just the last few years. New processing methods and new freezing methods allow foods to be kept as close to fresh as possible.

Tip

If you buy nonorganic veggies, take care to remove chemicals from the skin. Wash the vegetables in a full sink of water with a solution of 2 teaspoons of bleach and 1 tablespoon of dish detergent. There are also ready-made solutions available from health-food stores and mail-order catalogs.

Whole lines of organic and vegetarian foods are now being offered commercially, making it easier than ever before to bring a
wide variety of items to the consumer's table that might have
been difficult to find before. Still, I'm an old-fashioned guy. My
favorite foods are still fresh foods!

Stay Smart About Safety

According to a March 10, 1998, *New York Times* report, the federal
government is being urged by health officials to undertake new
and comprehensive efforts to detect cases of illness caused by
contaminated foods and to prevent future outbreaks.

If You Don't Have a Health-Food Store and Can't Find Organic Foods . . .

✔ Let your local supermarket manager know that you're inter-
ested in buying organic foods. Many chains have started to
stock organic produce, meat, and poultry as a matter of
course.

✔ Check out the frozen-food section of your supermarket.
There are many new variations on vegetarian and gluten-
free foods. They're not just in health-food stores anymore.

✔ Refer to the appendices of this book for information about
how you can order foods by mail.

The National Center for Health Statistics reported that food-
borne illnesses are among the leading reasons for emergency-
room visits each year. As an example, it was estimated that in a
one-year period between 1996 and 1997, the state of Minnesota's
4.4 million residents suffered 6.1 million diarrheal illnesses.

Although there are no firm numbers regarding the consumption of unsafe foods, botulism, staphylococcus, and toxoplas-
mosis are among the more common examples of fish-related

contamination. Viral hepatitis, caused by fecal contamination, unsafe mercury levels, and high levels of PCBs are potential hazards of eating foods from polluted water supplies. As with any animal product, bacterial and parasitic contamination are always possible. Alarmingly, fish is not subject to the same level of federal inspection as meat and poultry. Rather, a voluntary program of inspection is maintained by wholesale distributors and processors. It wasn't until 1991 that the Food and Drug Administration created a unit to monitor the safety of seafood!

Although the United States has long been touted as having the world's safest and least expensive food supply, it is becoming less so. A tremendous amount of our nation's food supply pours in from countries without even the minimal safeguards we employ to ensure food safety. An increasing number of food-borne illnesses, in fact, closely resemble what was once considered classic traveler's diarrhea. In other words, Montezuma's Revenge no longer requires luggage, merely a trip to the local supermarket.

Don't assume that you can relax your guard when you shop in a health-food store. Many health-food stores, especially the smaller ones, do not have the rapid turnover of a busy greengrocer or supermarket. Check the "sell by" dates on every package.

Know Your Organics

Commercial markets are stocking organic produce on a regular basis, a fairly recent innovation. Most of the organic produce and fruits are from California, a state with specific laws concerning the use of the word *organic*. In some markets, organic vegetables and fruits are displayed side by side with the nonorganic produce. In many instances, they're priced identically! I suspect that market demand will continue to push more and more vegetable and fruit growers back to the organic methods of cultivation. The cost of commercial fertilizers and pesticides will eventually make the nonorganic produce more expensive to grow. Despite the old pro and con arguments about the use of pesticides, it simply comes down to this piece of common sense:

No amount of pesticides, however small, has ever been discovered to be beneficial to the human body. Conversely, it is best to remember that organic fruits and vegetables bruise easily and spoil rapidly. Many areas of the world couldn't sustain sufficient levels of food production at this point without using pesticides. That's the paradox.

Pragmatically, a good rule of thumb is to purchase organic vegetables in preference to nonorganic vegetables if they're not exorbitantly priced. They taste better and are healthier for you. However, if you don't have a lot of money to spend and can't find reasonably priced organic produce, improvise. Fresh, high-quality nonorganic produce will be fine. The important thing is to eat plenty of fruits and vegetables. Organic or commercial, the valuable nutrients are there for the eating.

Make Your Kitchen Blood Type Friendly

YOU'LL FIND IT easier and more convenient to stock your kitchen with the staples that are right for your type. If you have more than one blood type in your household, mark your bins and containers accordingly.

Herbal Tea

STAPLE	PURCHASING	STORING
TYPE O		
Cayenne		
Chickweed		Can keep for 1 year
Dandelion		
Fenugreek		
Ginger		
Hops		
Linden		
Mulberry		
Parsley		
Peppermint		
Rose hips		
Sarsaparilla		
Slippery elm		
TYPE A		
Alfalfa		
Aloe		
Burdock		
Chamomile		
Echinacea		
Fenugreek		
Ginger		
Ginseng		
Green tea		
Hawthorn		
Milk thistle		
Rose hips		
St.-John's-wort		
Slippery elm		
Valerian		

STAPLE	PURCHASING	STORING
TYPE B		
Ginger		
Ginseng		
Green tea		
Licorice		
Parsley		
Peppermint		
Raspberry leaf		
Rose hips		
Sage		
TYPE AB		
Alfalfa		
Burdock		
Chamomile		
Echinacea		
Ginger		
Ginseng		
Green tea		
Hawthorn		
Licorice root		
Rose hips		
Strawberry leaf		

Spices/Condiments

STAPLE	PURCHASING	STORING
TYPE O		
Carob		
Cayenne pepper		

STAPLE	PURCHASING	STORING
TYPE O (continued)		
Curry		
Dulse		Can be stored indefi-
Ginger		nitely (the dry ones)
Horseradish		
Parsley		
Miso		
Tamari		Up to 4 months
Turmeric		
TYPE A		
Garlic		
Ginger		
Miso		
Mustard seed		
Soy Sauce		
Tamari		
TYPE B		
Cayenne pepper		
Curry		
Ginger		
Nori		
Horseradish		
Parsley		
TYPE AB		
Curry		
Garlic		
Horseradish		
Kelp		
Miso		
Parsley		

Sweeteners

STAPLE	PURCHASING	STORING
TYPE O		
Brown rice syrup		
Honey*		Will keep indefinitely
Maple syrup		if stored appropriately.
Molasses		
Sugar in the raw		
TYPE A		
Barley malt		
Brown rice syrup		
Brown sugar		
Honey*		
Maple syrup		
Molasses		
Sugar in the raw		
TYPE B		
Apple butter		
Brown sugar		
Honey*		
Molasses		
Sugar in the raw		
TYPE AB		
Honey*		
Molasses		
Sugar in the raw		

*Honey should not be fed to children under one year of age
as it may cause botulism in small babies.*

Vinegars, Sauces, & Oils

STAPLE	PURCHASING	STORING
TYPE O		
Linseed (flaxseed oil)		Can be stored
Olive oil		indefinitely if the
Tamari		lids are on properly.
Canola oil		
Sesame oil		
TYPE A		
Linseed (flaxseed oil)		
Mustard		
Olive oil		
Soy sauce		
Tamari		
TYPE B		
Horseradish		
Olive oil		
TYPE AB		
Canola oil		
Miso		
Olive oil		

Grains

STAPLE	PURCHASING	STORING
TYPE O		
Kasha	Grocery stores,	Best way to store is in
Millet	health-food	freezer or refrigerator.
Quinoa	stores, and mail	Whole grains will keep
Rye	order	for several months if
Spelt berries		stored in an airtight
Spelt		container in a cool, dry
		place.
TYPE A		
Amaranth		Rice will keep 3 to 6
Buckwheat kasha		months if stored
Millet		properly (airtight
Oats		container in cool,
Rice		dry place).
Rice pasta		
Soba noodles		
TYPE B		
Basmati rice		Cooled rice will only
Brown rice		keep for a few days in
Millet		the refrigerator. Cooled
Oats		rice can be frozen.
Quinoa		Quinoa can be stored 3
Spelt berries		to 6 months in the
		refrigerator.
TYPE AB		
Basmati rice		
Brown rice		
Millet		
Oats		
Spelt berries		

STAPLE	PURCHASING	STORING
TYPE AB (continued)		
White rice		
Wild rice		
Watch for insect infestation!		

Flour

STAPLE	PURCHASING	STORING
TYPE O		
Rye flour Spelt (white/ whole-grain)	Health-food store, mail order, grocery stores (selected)	Whole-grain flour should be stored in an airtight container in a cool, dry place or in the refrigerator. Flour can be kept up to six months.
TYPE A		
Amaranth Brown rice Oat flour Quinoa Rice flour Rye flour Soy powder Spelt (white/ whole-grain)	Health-food store, mail order, grocery stores (selected)	

STAPLE	PURCHASING	STORING
TYPE B		
Oat bran	Health-food	
Soy powder (pow-	store, mail order,	
dered protein)	grocery stores	
Spelt (white/	(selected)	
whole-grain)		
TYPE AB		
Oat flour	Health-food	
Rice flour	store, mail order,	
Rye flour	grocery stores	
Soy powder	(selected)	
Spelt (white/		
whole-grain)		
Sprouted wheat flour		

Watch for insect infestation!

Cereals

STAPLE	PURCHASING	STORING
TYPE O		
Amaranth	Health-food	Cereals should be kept
Cream of Rice	stores, some	in an airtight container
Puffed rice	grocery stores	away from heat and
Spelt		moisture. Storing them
		in the refrigerator or in
		a cool place (40 degrees
		F) delays rancidity and
		the development of
		mold and helps to pre-
		vent insect infestation.
		Cereals can be stored
		up to six months.

STAPLE	PURCHASING	STORING
TYPE A		
Amaranth	Health-food stores,	
Buckwheat	some grocery stores	
Kasha		
Oat bran		
Oatmeal		
Spelt		
TYPE B		
Millet	Health-food stores,	
Oat bran	some grocery stores	
Oatmeal		
Puffed rice		
Rice bran		
Spelt		
TYPE AB		
Millet	Health-food stores,	
Oat bran	some grocery stores	
Oatmeal		
Puffed rice		
Rice bran		
Spelt		

Pasta

STAPLE	PURCHASING	STORING
TYPE O		
Quinoa	Grocery store,	Fresh pasta will last 1 to
Rice pasta	health-food	2 days in the refrigera-
Spelt pasta	store, mail order	tor and can be frozen
		up to 1 month. Pre-
		packaged pasta can be
		stored up to 6 months.

STAPLE	PURCHASING	STORING
TYPE A		
Artichoke pasta		
Quinoa		
Soba noodles		
Spelt pasta		
TYPE B		
Quinoa		
Rice pasta		
Spinach pasta		
TYPE AB		
Quinoa		
Rice pasta		

Seeds/Nuts

STAPLE	PURCHASING	STORING
TYPE O		
Pumpkin seeds	Grocery store,	Nuts should be stored
Walnuts	health-food	in an airtight container
	store, mail order	in a cool, dry place.
		Unshelled nuts can be
		stored up to 8 months.
		Shelled nuts should be
		used within 3 months
		of purchasing.
TYPE A		
Peanut butter		
Peanuts		
Pumpkin seeds		

STAPLE	PURCHASING	STORING
TYPE B		
Almonds		
Walnuts		
TYPE AB		
Chestnuts		
Peanut butter		
Peanuts		
Walnuts		

Beans/Legumes

STAPLE	PURCHASING	STORING
TYPE O		
Adzuki beans	Health-food	Legumes can be stored
Black-eyed peas	stores, selected	in an airtight container
Pinto beans	grocery stores,	in a cool, dry place up
	mail order. When	to 1 year.
	purchasing, look	
	for legumes that	
	are firm, brightly	
	colored, and uni-	
	form in size	
TYPE A		
Adzuki beans		
Black beans		
Black-eyed peas		
Green beans		
Lentils—domestic		
Lentils—green		
Lentils—red		

STAPLE	PURCHASING	STORING
TYPE A (continued)		
Pinto beans		
Red soy beans		
TYPE B		
Kidney beans		
Lima beans		
Navy beans		
Red soy beans		
TYPE AB		
Lentils—green		
Navy beans		
Pinto beans		
Red beans		
Red soy beans		

In the Kitchen

Preparing Fish and Meats

Most of the nutritional value of food can be lost by improper preparation. This is especially true of high-protein animal foods such as meats and fish. I ask those of my patients who eat meat as part of their Blood Type Diet to take a couple of extra steps before cooking any meats. First, I ask them to remove any excess skin or fat from the meat. Second, boil water in a pot large enough to hold the meat, turn off the heat, and just let the meat soak in the water three to five minutes. I know this sounds distressing. Won't the meat be ruined? Actually, this won't alter the flavor or texture, but it will remove any chemicals that have resulted from the oxidation of the meat's surface. It will also kill any bacteria that may have developed from improper handling. A caution, however: If the piece of meat you're treating is at all suspect in terms of freshness, placing it in the hot water won't make it any more edible. If meat is spoiled or tainted in any way, discard it. The same treatment should be given to fish.

Frying, Smoking, Curing, Pickling

Fried, smoked, cured, or pickled meats or fish should be avoided by all blood types. Although many cultures favor the flavors produced by deep frying, dangerous carcinogens are produced in the process. The effects of eating fried foods on the heart and cardiovascular system are well documented.

Smoked or cured meats and fish, such as cold cuts, hot dogs, ham, and bacon as well as smoked salmon and pickled herring, contain undesirable levels of nitrates and nitrites as well as high levels of sodium. Nitrates have been linked to stomach cancer, a disease which Type Os, Type As, and Type ABs are prone to: Type O because of high stomach-acid levels, and Type A and Type AB because of their low stomach acid.

Stir Frying

Stir frying is a lot healthier than deep frying. Certainly less oil is used. The concept of stir frying involves cooking food at a high temperature in a searingly hot pan. This quickly seals in the food's flavors in a crisply textured manner. Meat, fish, tofu, and vegetables can be stir fried using a deep, cone-shaped wok, designed to concentrate the heat in a small area at its base. This allows small amounts of food to be cooked there and then moved to the cooler upper edges of the pan. Cook the meats and vegetables that require a longer time first, then move them to the upper edges of the pan. Then add the vegetables that require less cooking to the base of the wok. The idea is to keep all of the food hot and cooking, but at different times and at different degrees. Skillful stir frying can add a lot of taste and enjoyment to a few vegetables and a little meat, fish, or tofu.

> ### Tip
>
> Stir frying is an especially effective way to cook tofu. As it cooks, tofu absorbs the flavors of other ingredients—a bit of garlic or ginger mixed in with the vegetables will enhance the flavor even more. For people who are not accustomed to eating tofu, stir frying is a good way to start.

Broiling, Poaching, Parboiling, and Baking

Broiling generates some carcinogenic materials, but it is generally healthier than frying. If meats are lean and the cooking time is limited to simply "browning" the surface, it should not cause any problems. Baking, poaching, and parboiling are safe methods of cooking that are usually best used for foods such as fish filets or eggs, which require only a short amount of time to cook thoroughly.

Steaming

Steaming is the most delicious way I know to prepare a host of vegetables. It's a quick and effective method of cooking that keeps the nutrients in the food. Boiling leaves most of the nutrients in the water. A simple steamer basket can be purchased at most supermarkets and at almost any hardware or department store. The basket sits inside a large pot filled with a shallow amount of water below the level of the basket. Add vegetables, cover, and heat. Crisp broccoli takes about five or six minutes; Brussels sprouts a while longer. The most important thing to remember about steaming is that all of the nutrients in the vegetable find their way to you. None of the flavor or goodness of the food is lost in the cooking process. The food has merely been made more assimilable.

Pots, Pans, Utensils

It can be dangerous to use the wrong kind of pot or pan for cooking. Never use decorative-type pots and pans for cooking, such as copper or pewter pans. Some are made of a mixture of lead and silver, toxic metals that can leach into the food during the cooking process. Also be especially careful with ceramic pots. Make sure the glazes and paints are free of lead. Porcelain, Corning-type glassware, and enameled surfaces are fine for cooking.

Cast-iron skillets, which allow small amounts of iron to get into the food, are generally safe, and probably provided an important source of iron in the old days. Make sure that any rust or corrosion that has built up on the surface of the pan is thoroughly removed with an abrasive, such as steel wool.

Aluminum cookware is very inexpensive and still commonly used and sold. I believe there's a real potential health problem with using aluminum for cooking. Aluminum is not easily removed from the body, and the one characteristic common to all people who suffer from Alzheimer's disease is that they have an inordinately high accumulation of aluminum in their brain tissue. Aluminum is a soft metal that is easily transferred to food by spoons and ladles made of harder metals. Aluminum also reacts with acids in the foods, which can result in the binding and loss of vitamin C content.

Stainless steel is your safest choice for pots and pans. The metal is hard and virtually inert. In other words, none of it will transfer to your food during the cooking process. Some stainless-steel cookware is "aluminum-clad" on the bottom to create a surface which acts as a heat conductor. This is fine, as the aluminum is bonded to the outside of the pot and cannot react with the food inside. Most Teflon-coated cooking surfaces eventually become scratched unless you are careful about washing and drying. If you do use Teflon-coated cookware, always use soft plastic tools when cooking to avoid scratching the surface. Some of the latest Teflon-like surfaces are harder and therefore much safer.

Recommended Kitchen Tools

TOOL	ALTERNATIVES	USES	ADVANTAGES
Stainless-steel cookware		All	Safe
Cast-iron pans			Excellent heat conductors
Cast-iron coated with enamel			Excellent heat conductors
Wok	Cast-iron pan Skillet	Stir-fry	Wok enables rapid cooking over very high heat
Large 10" skillet	Wok	Sauté Steam Frittata Omelets Stir-fry	
Good set of Revere Ware			Long-lasting
Wooden spoons			Quiet
Stainless-steel spoons, ladles, etc.			Safe
Measuring cups/spoons			
Whisk			
Best knives one can afford 8" chef 6" chef boring paring slicing serrated for bread			If cared for, they will last a lifetime
Stainless-steel steamer		For vegetables	Better than boiling vegetables
Stainless-steel grater		Cheese Vegetables	

TOOL	ALTERNATIVES	USES	ADVANTAGES
Set of mixing bowls			
Small & large colanders			
Blender			Food processor
Bread machine (2-lb.)			
Food processor	Blender	Drinks Sauces Dressings	

At the Table

THERE'S MORE TO eating than the food you put into your system. The digestive process is truly holistic. You might be surprised about the elements that have a practical impact on the way your body utilizes foods. To make the most of your meal, heed the following:

1. Don't drink with your meal.

The first time Martha visited my father's house before we were married, she was surprised to find no water glasses on the table. My father discovered many years ago that consuming liquids with food dilutes the digestive juices. You'll notice that we include beverages with the blood type menus. However, try to drink them separately from the meal itself. For example, have a glass of wine a half hour before dinner and drink your tea or coffee a half hour after dinner.

2. Leave your tension at the door.

According to a Roman proverb, the secret to healing is "Dr. Diet, Dr. Quiet, and Dr. Happy." If you eat when you're nervous or tense, your stress hormones produce too many digestive juices, which leads to heartburn and acid stomach. The dinner hour is not the time to discuss Johnny's failing report card.

3. Stop talking.

In addition to the obvious connection between talking and stress, there's a very practical reason why meals should be silent. When you talk, you tend to swallow large amounts of air, and that causes gas. Talking also interferes with the chewing process, and food must be well chewed in order to be digested properly. The old parental reminder "Don't talk with your mouth full" is a good rule of thumb, and not just for etiquette reasons.

4. Chew your food.

People who bolt their food down as if they're in some kind of contest deprive themselves of one of life's greatest pleasures— eating and enjoying the flavors, aromas, colors, and textures of their food. The importance of mastication—using your teeth, lips, gums, and mouth to thoroughly chew and break down what- ever it is that you're eating—can't be emphasized enough. Be- cause the secretion of gastric juices is initiated by the sense of taste, chewing thoroughly and keeping the food in your mouth long enough to fully extract its full flavor helps prepare the stom- ach for proper digestion. This is also why foods should be eaten in their natural state. Digestive enzymes react only on the sur- face of food particles, not on their interior, so the rate of digestion depends upon the total surface area exposed to gastric and in- testinal secretions. The more you chew the food, the greater the surface area, and the more effective the digestion throughout the gastrointestinal tract. This, in turn, increases the ease with which food is passed from the stomach to the small intestines and other areas of the body, thereby placing less strain on the digestive system.

If your diet includes meats and seafood, you must take the time to thoroughly chew them, even up to thirty times per bite. Because starches such as bread, potatoes, and fruit begin the process of digestion right in the mouth, they need to be thoroughly chewed to facilitate that breakdown. In addition to expediting proper digestion, thorough chewing also eases elimination because it warms the food, and this accelerates the catalytic activities of the enzymes. Swallowing cold foods whole slows the digestive process by inhibiting the proper secretion of enzymes.

The recipes and menus that we have developed for you reinforce the philosophy that eating well is a restorative, energizing, and almost mystical experience. Let's all eat in happiness and good health.

Understanding Food Combining

When you can, try to keep meats and seafood away from dense starches, such as potatoes and grains. Combining starches and proteins is a favorite of many people, especially in the form of sandwiches, which are a quick, convenient, and portable meal. It's okay to eat sandwiches sometimes—we even offer some delicious and healthy variations in this book.

The word *sandwich* originated with Lord Sandwich, an English noble who asked that his meat be placed between two pieces of bread, so that he could remain at the gambling table. Are you using this sort of thinking to decide what to eat? Stuffing a sandwich down your throat during a fifteen-minute lunch break almost guarantees a feeling of lethargy. It's also a quick path to gas, bloating, and other intestinal problems. Paying attention to which foods you eat together is important, as proteins and carbohydrates digest at different rates.

O, A, B, AB
Food
Charts

Type O Diet

FOOD GROUP *Portion*	FREQUENCY BY ANCESTRAL TYPE	HIGHLY BENEFICIAL
MEAT & POULTRY: *portion:* men 4–6 oz. women/ children 2–5 oz.	**WEEKLY** *Lean Red Meats:* Caucasians: 4–6X Africans: 5–7X Asians: 3–5X *Poultry:* Caucasians: 2–3X Africans: 1–2X Asians: 3–4X	beef, ground beef, buffalo, heart, lamb, liver, mutton, veal, venison
SEAFOOD: *portion:* 4–6 oz.	**WEEKLY** Caucasians: 3–5X Africans: 1–4X Asians: 4–6X	bluefish, cod, hake, halibut, herring, mackerel, pike, rainbow trout, red snapper, salmon, sardine, shad, sole, striped bass, sturgeon, swordfish, tilefish, whitefish, white perch, yel- low perch, yellowtail
EGGS & DAIRY: *portion:* egg: 1 cheeses: 2 oz. yogurt: 4–6 oz. milk: 4–6 oz.	**WEEKLY** *Eggs:* Caucasians: 3–4X Africans: 0X Asians: 5X *Cheeses:* Caucasians: 0–3X Africans: 0X Asians: 0–3X *Yogurt:* Caucasians: 0–3X Africans: 0X Asians: 0–3X *Milk:* Caucasians: 0–1X Africans: 0X Asians: 0–2X	none

NEUTRAL	AVOID
chicken, Cornish hens, duck, partridge, pheasant, quail, rabbit, turkey	bacon, goose, ham, pork
abalone, albacore (tuna), anchovy, beluga, bluegill bass, carp, clam, crab, crayfish, eel, flounder, frog, gray sole, grouper, haddock, lobster, mahimahi, monkfish, mussels, ocean perch, oysters, pickerel, porgy, sailfish, scallop, sea bass, sea trout, shark, shrimp, silver perch, smelt, snail, squid (calamari), turtle, weakfish	barracuda, catfish, caviar, conch, herring (pickled), lox (smoked salmon), octopus
butter, farmer, feta, goat cheese, mozzarella, soy cheese,* soy milk* *good dairy alternatives	American cheese, blue, Brie, buttermilk, Camembert, casein, Cheddar, Colby, cottage, cream cheese, Edam, Emmenthal, goat milk, Gouda, Gruyère, ice cream, Jarlsberg, kefir, Monterey Jack, Munster, Parmesan, provolone, neufchatel, ricotta, skim or 2% milk, string cheese, Swiss, whey, whole milk, yogurt (all varieties)

Type O Diet

FOOD GROUP Portion	FREQUENCY BY ANCESTRAL TYPE	HIGHLY BENEFICIAL
OILS & FATS: *portion:* 1 tablespoon	**WEEKLY** Caucasians: 4–8X Africans: 1–5X Asians: 3–7X	linseed (flaxseed) oil, olive oil
NUTS & SEEDS: *portion:* nuts & seeds: 6–8 nuts nut butters: 1 tablespoon	**WEEKLY** *Nuts & Seeds:* Caucasians: 3–4X Africans: 2–5X Asians: 2–3X *Nut Butters:* Caucasians: 3–7X Africans: 3–4X Asians: 2–4X	pumpkin seeds, walnuts
BEANS & LEGUMES: *portion:* 1 cup dry	**WEEKLY** Caucasians: 1–2X Africans: 1–2X Asians: 2–6X	adzuki beans, pinto beans, black-eyed peas
CEREALS: *portion:* 1 cup dry	**WEEKLY** Caucasians: 2–3X Africans: 2–3X Asians: 2–4X	none
BREADS & MUFFINS: *portion:* 1 slice bread or cracker 1 muffin	**DAILY** *Breads/ Crackers:* Caucasians: 0–2X Africans: 0–4X Asians: 0–4X *Muffins:* Caucasians: 0–1X Africans: 0–2X Asians: 0–1X	Essene bread, Ezekial bread
GRAINS & PASTA: *portion:* grains:1 cup dry pastas:1 cup dry	**WEEKLY** All Ancestral Types *Grains:* 0–3X *Pastas:* 0–3X	none

NEUTRAL	AVOID
canola oil, cod liver oil, sesame oil	corn oil, cottonseed oil, peanut oil, safflower oil
almond butter, almonds, chestnuts, filberts, hickory nuts, macadamias, pecans, pignoli (pine), sesame butter (tahini), sesame seeds, sunflower butter, sunflower seeds	Brazil, cashew, litchi, peanuts, peanut butter, pistachios, poppy seeds
black beans, broad beans, cannellini beans, fava beans, garbanzo beans, green beans, jicama beans, lima beans, northern beans, red beans, red soy beans, snap beans, string beans, white beans, green peas, pea pods	copper beans, kidney beans, navy beans, tamarind beans, domestic lentils, green lentils, red lentils
amaranth, barley, buckwheat, Cream of Rice, kamut, kasha, puffed millet, puffed rice, rice bran, spelt	cornflakes, cornmeal, Cream of Wheat, Familia, farina, Grape Nuts, oat bran, oatmeal, seven grain, shredded wheat, wheat bran, wheat germ
brown-rice bread, Fin crisp, gluten-free bread, Ideal flat bread, millet, rice cakes, 100% rye bread, rye crisps, Rye Vita, soy-flour bread, spelt bread, Wasa bread	wheat bagels, corn muffins, durum wheat, English muffins, high-protein bread, wheat matzoh, multigrain bread, oat-bran bread, pumpernickel, sprouted-wheat bread, wheat-bran muffins, whole-wheat bread
barley flour, buckwheat, kasha, artichoke pasta, quinoa, basmati rice, brown rice, white rice, wild rice, rice flour, rye flour, spelt flour	bulgur-wheat flour, couscous flour, durum-wheat flour, gluten flour, graham flour, oat flour, soba noodles, semolina pasta, spinach pasta, sprouted-wheat flour, white flour, whole-wheat flour

Type O Diet

FOOD GROUP *Portion*	FREQUENCY BY ANCESTRAL TYPE	HIGHLY BENEFICIAL
VEGETABLES: *portion:* raw, cooked, or steamed: 1 cup prepared	**DAILY** All Ancestral Types *Raw vegetables:* 3–5X *Cooked or* *steamed* *vegetables:* 3–5X	artichokes (Jerusalem & domestic), beet leaves, broccoli, chicory, collard greens, dandelion, escarole, garlic, horseradish, kale, kohlrabi, leek, romaine lettuce, okra, red onions, Spanish onions, yellow onions, parsley, parsnips, red peppers, sweet potatoes, pumpkin, seaweed, spinach, Swiss chard, turnips
FRUITS: *portion:* 1 fruit or 3–5 oz.	**DAILY** All Ancestral Types 3–4X	dried or fresh figs, dark plums, red plums, green plums, prunes
JUICES & **FLUIDS:** *portion:* juices: 8 oz. water: 8 oz.	**DAILY** All Ancestral Types Juices: 2–3X Water: 4–7X	black cherry, pineapple, prune

NEUTRAL	AVOID
arugula, asparagus, bamboo shoots, beets, bok choy, caraway, carrots, celery, chervil, coriander, cucumber, daikon, dill, endive, fennel, fiddlehead ferns, ginger, bibb lettuce, Boston lettuce, iceberg lettuce, mesclun lettuce, lima beans, abalone, enoki mushrooms, Portobello mushrooms, tree oyster mushrooms, green olives, green onions, green peppers, jalapeño peppers, yellow peppers, radicchio, radishes, rappini, rutabaga, scallion, shallots, snow peas, mung sprouts, radish sprouts, all types squash, tempeh, tofu, tomato, water chestnut, watercress, yams, zucchini	avocado, Chinese cabbage, red cabbage, white cabbage, cauliflower, white corn, yellow corn, eggplant, domestic mushrooms, shiitake mushrooms, mustard greens, black olives, Greek olives, Spanish olives, red potatoes, white potatoes, alfalfa sprouts, Brussels sprouts
apples, apricots, bananas, blueberries, boysenberries, cherries, cranberries, black & red currants, red dates, elderberries, gooseberries, grapefruit, black grapes, concord grapes, green grapes, red grapes, guava, kiwi, kumquat, lemons, limes, loganberries, mangoes, canang melon, casaba melon, Crenshaw melon, Christmas melon, Spanish melon, watermelon, nectarines, papayas, peaches, pears, persimmons, pineapples, pomegranates, prickly pears, raisins, rasberries, starfruit (carambola)	blackberries, coconuts, cantaloupe melon, honeydew melon, oranges, plantains, rhubarb, strawberries, tangerines
apricot, carrot, celery, cranberry, cucumber, grape, grapefruit, papaya, tomato water (with lemon), vegetable juice	apple, apple cider, cabbage, orange

Type O Diet

FOOD GROUP *Portion*	FREQUENCY BY ANCESTRAL TYPE	HIGHLY BENEFICIAL
SPICES:		Carob, cayenne pepper, curry, dulse, kelp (bladderwrack), parsley, turmeric
CONDIMENTS:		none
HERBAL TEAS:		cayenne, chickweed, dandelion, fenugreek, ginger, hops, linden, mulberry, parsley, peppermint, rose hips, sarsaparilla, slippery elm
MISC. BEVERAGES:		seltzer water

NEUTRAL	AVOID
agar, allspice, almond extract, anise, arrowroot, barley malt, basil, bay leaf, bergamot, brown-rice syrup, cardamon, chervil, chives, chocolate, clove, coriander, cream of tartar, cumin, dill, garlic, plain gelatin, honey, horseradish, maple syrup, marjoram, mint, miso, molasses, dry mustard, paprika, peppercorns, pepper, red pepper flakes, peppermint, pimiento, rice syrup, rosemary, saffron, sage, salt, savory, soy sauce, spearmint, sucanat, white & brown sugar, tamari, tamarind, tapioca, tarragon, thyme, wintergreen	capers, cinnamon, cornstarch, corn syrup, nutmeg, ground black pepper, white pepper, vanilla extract, apple cider vinegar, balsamic, red wine vinegar, white vinegar
apple butter, jam & jelly from acceptable fruits, mustard, salad dressing (low-fat from acceptable ingredients), Worcestershire sauce	ketchup, mayonnaise, dill pickles, kosher pickles, sweet pickles, sour pickles, relish
catnip, chamomile, dong quai, elder, ginseng, green tea, hawthorn, horehound, licorice root, mullein, rasberry leaf, sage, skullcap, spearmint, thyme, valerian, vervain, white birch, white oak bark, yarrow	alfalfa, aloe, burdock, coltsfoot, corn silk, echinacea, gentian, goldenseal, red clover, rhubarb, St.-John's-wort, senna, shepherd's purse, strawberry leaf, yellow dock
beer, green tea, red wine, white wine	regular & decaf coffee, distilled liquors, cola, diet cola & other sodas, black teas (regular & decaf)

Type A Diet

FOOD GROUP *Portion*	FREQUENCY BY ANCESTRAL TYPE		HIGHLY BENEFICIAL
MEAT & **POULTRY:** *portion:* men 4–6 oz. women/- children 2–5 oz.	**WEEKLY** *Lean red meats:* Caucasians: 0X Africans: 0–1X Asians 0–1X *Poultry:* Caucasians: 0–3X Africans: 0–3X Asians: 1–4X		none
SEAFOOD: *portion:* 4–6 oz.	**WEEKLY** Caucasians: 1–4X Africans: 0–3X Asians: 1–4X		carp, cod, grouper, mackerel, monk- fish, pickerel, red snapper, rainbow trout, salmon, sardine, sea trout, silver perch, snail, whitefish, yellow perch
EGGS & **DAIRY:** *portion:* egg: 1 cheeses: 2 oz. yogurt: 4–6 oz. milk: 4–6 oz.	**WEEKLY** *Eggs:* Caucasians: 1–3X Africans: 1–3X Asians: 1–3X *Cheeses:* Caucasians: 2–4X Africans: 1–3X Asians: 0X *Yogurt:* Caucasians: 1–3X Africans: 0X Asians: 0–3X *Milk:* Caucasians: 0–4X Africans: 0X Asians: 0X		soya cheese,* soy milk* *good dairy alternative
OILS & FATS: *portion:* 1 tablespoon	**WEEKLY** Caucasians: 2–6X Africans: 3–8X Asians: 2–6X		linseed (flaxseed) oil, olive oil

NEUTRAL	AVOID
chicken, Cornish hens, turkey	bacon, beef, ground beef, buffalo, duck, goose, ham, heart, lamb, liver, mutton, partridge, pheasant, pork, quail, rabbit, veal, venison
abalone, albacore (tuna), mahimahi, ocean perch, pike, porgy, sailfish, sea bass, shark, smelt, snapper, sturgeon, swordfish, weakfish, white perch, yellowtail	anchovy, barracuda, beluga, bluefish, bluegill bass, catfish, caviar, clam, conch, crab, crayfish, eel, flounder, frog, gray sole, haddock, hake, halibut, herring, lobster, lox (smoked salmon), mussels, octopus, oysters, scallop, shad, shrimp, sole, squid (calamari), striped bass, tilefish, turtle
farmer, feta, goat cheese, goat's milk, kefir, mozzarella (low-fat), ricotta (low fat), string cheese, yogurt with fruit, frozen yogurt	American cheese, blue, Brie, butter, buttermilk, Camembert, casein, Cheddar, colby, cottage, cream cheese, Edam, Emmenthal, Gouda, Gruyère, ice cream, Jarlsberg, Monterey Jack, Munster, neufchatel, Parmesan, provolone, sherbet, skim or 2% milk, Swiss, whey, whole milk
canola oil, cod liver oil	corn oil, cottonseed oil, peanut oil, safflower oil, sesame oil

Type A Diet

FOOD GROUP *Portion*	FREQUENCY BY ANCESTRAL TYPE	HIGHLY BENEFICIAL

**NUTS &
SEEDS:**
portion:
nuts & seeds:
  small handful
nut butters:
  1 tablespoon
	WEEKLY
	Nuts & Seeds:
	Caucasians: 2–5X
	Africans: 4–6X
	Asians: 4–6X
	Nut Butters:
	Caucasians: 1–4X
	Africans: 3–5X
	Asians: 2–4X
		peanuts, peanut butter, pumpkin seeds

BEANS & LEGUMES: *portion:* 1 cup dry	**WEEKLY** Caucasians: 3–6X Africans: 4–7X Asians: 2–5X	adzuki beans, black beans, green beans, pinto beans, red soy beans, lentils (domestic, red & green), black- eyed peas
CEREALS: *portion:* whole grain: 1 cup dry	**WEEKLY** *Whole Grains:* Caucasians: 5–9X Africans: 6–10X Asians: 4–8X	amaranth, kasha

**GRAINS &
PASTAS:**
portion:
grains:
  1 cup dry
pastas:
  1 cup dry
	WEEKLY
	Grains
	Caucasians: 2–4X
	Africans: 2–3X
	Asians: 2–4X
	Pastas:
	Caucasians: 2–4X
	Africans: 2–3X
	Asians: 2–4X
		kasha, oat flour, rice flour, rye flour,
		soba noodles, artichoke pasta

**BREADS &
MUFFINS:**
portion:
  1 slice bread
  or crackers
  1 muffin
	DAILY
	*Breads &
	Crackers:*
	Caucasians: 3–5X
	Africans: 2–4X
	Asians: 2–4X
	Muffins:
	Caucasians: 1–2X
	Africans: 1X
	Asians: 1X
		Essene bread, Ezekiel bread, soya-flour
		bread, sprouted-wheat bread, rice
		cakes

NEUTRAL	AVOID
almond butter, almonds, chestnuts, filberts, hickory, litchis, macadamias, pignoli (pine), poppy seeds, sesame seeds, sesame butter, sunflower butter, sunflower seeds, walnuts	Brazil, cashews, pistachios
broad beans, cannellini beans, fava beans, jicama beans, snap beans, string beans, white beans, green peas, pea pods, snow peas	copper beans, garbanzo beans, kidney beans, lima beans, navy beans, red beans, tamarind beans
barley, cornflakes, cornmeal, Cream of Rice, kamut, puffed millet, oat bran, oatmeal, puffed rice, rice bran, spelt	Cream of Wheat, Familia, farina, granola, Grape Nuts, seven grain, shredded wheat, wheat bran, wheat germ
couscous, barley flour, bulgur wheat flour, durum-wheat flour, gluten flour, graham flour, sprouted-wheat flour, spelt noodles, quinoa, basmati rice, brown rice, white rice, wild rice	white flour, whole-wheat flour, semolina pasta, spinach pasta
brown-rice bread, corn muffins, Fin crisp, gluten-free bread, Ideal flat bread, millet, oat bran muffins, 100% rye bread, rye crisps, Rye Vita, spelt bread, Wasa bread	durum wheat, high-protein bread, multigrain bread, English muffins, pumpernickel wheat-bran muffins, whole-wheat bread, wheat matzoh

Type A Diet

FOOD GROUP *Portion*	FREQUENCY BY ANCESTRAL TYPE	HIGHLY BENEFICIAL
VEGETABLE: *portion:* raw: 1 cup cooked: 1 cup cooked soy products: 6–8 oz.	**DAILY** *Raw Vegetables:* Caucasians: 2–5X Africans: 3–6X Asians: 2–5X *Cooked* *Vegetables:* Caucasians: 3–6X Africans: 1–4X Asians: 3–6X **WEEKLY** *Soy Products:* Caucasians: 4–6X Africans: 4–6X Asians: 5–7X	alfalfa sprouts, domestic artichokes, Jerusalem artichokes, beet leaves, broccoli, carrots, chicory, collard greens, dandelion, escarole, garlic, horseradish, kale, kohlrabi, leek, romaine lettuce, okra, red Spanish onions, yellow onions, parsley, parsnips, pumpkin, spinach, Swiss chard, tempeh, tofu, turnips
FRUITS: *portion:* 1 fruit or 3–5 oz.	**DAILY** All Ancestral Types 3–4X	apricots, blackberries, blueberries, boysenberries, cherries, cranberries, dried figs, fresh figs, grapefruit, lemons, pineapple, dark plums, green plums, red plums, prunes
JUICES & **FLUIDS:** *portion:* 8 oz.	**DAILY** All Ancestral Types *Juices:* 4–5X *Lemon & Water:* 1X in morning *Water:* 1–3X	apricots, carrots, celery, black cherries, grapefruit, pineapple, prunes, water with lemon

NEUTRAL	AVOID
arugula, asparagus, avocado, bamboo shoots, beets, bok choy, caraway, cauliflower, celery, chervil, coriander, white & yellow corn, cucumber, daikon radish, endive, fennel, fiddlehead ferns, bibb lettuce, Boston lettuce, iceberg lettuce, mesclun lettuce, abalone mushrooms, enoki mushrooms, maitaki mushrooms, shiitake mushrooms, Portobello mushrooms, tree oyster mushrooms, mustard greens, green olives, green onions, radicchio, radishes, rappini, rutabaga, scallion, seaweed, shallots, Brussels sprouts, mung sprouts, radish sprouts, all types squash, water chestnut, watercress, zucchini	Chinese cabbage, red cabbage, white cabbage, eggplant, lima beans, domestic mushrooms, black olives, Greek olives, Spanish olives, green peppers, jalapeño peppers, red peppers, yellow peppers, sweet potatoes, red potatoes, white potatoes, tomatoes, yams
apples, black currants, red currants, dates, elderberries, gooseberries, grapes (black, Concord, green & red), guava, kiwi, kumquat, limes, loganberries, canang melon, casaba melon, Christmas melon, Crenshaw melon, muskmelon, Spanish melon, watermelon, nectarines, peaches, pears, persimmons, pomegranates, prickly pears, raisins, raspberries, star fruit, strawberries	bananas, coconuts, mangoes, cantaloupe, honeydew melon, oranges, papayas, plantains, rhubarb, tangerines
apple, apple cider, cabbage, cucumber, cranberry, grape, vegetable juice (corresponding to highlighted vegetables)	orange, papaya, tomato

Type A Diet

FOOD GROUP *Portion*	FREQUENCY BY ANCESTRAL TYPE	HIGHLY BENEFICIAL
SPICES		barley malt, blackstrap molasses, garlic, ginger, miso, soy sauce, tamari sauce
CONDIMENTS		mustard
HERBAL TEAS		alfalfa, aloe, burdock, chamomile, echinacea, fenugreek, ginger, ginseng, green tea, hawthorn, milk thistle, rose hips, St.-John's-wort, slippery elm, stone root, valerian
MISC. BEVERAGES		coffee (regular & decaf), green tea, red wine

NEUTRAL	AVOID
agar, allspice, almond extract, anise, arrowroot, basil, bay leaf, bergamot, brown-rice syrup, cardamom, carob, chervil, chives, chocolate, cinnamon, cloves, coriander, cornstarch, corn syrup, cream of tartar, cumin, curry, dill, dulse, honey, horseradish, kelp, maple syrup, marjoram, mint, dry mustard, nutmeg, oregano, paprika, parsley, peppermint, pimiento, rice syrup, rosemary, saffron, sage, salt, savory, spearmint, brown sugar, white sugar, tamarind, tapioca, tarragon, thyme, turmeric, vanilla extract	capers, plain gelatin, ground black pepper, cayenne pepper, peppercorn pepper, red pepper flakes, white pepper, apple cider vinegar, red wine vinegar, balsamic vinegar, white vinegar, wintergreen
jam & jelly (from acceptable fruits), salad dressing (low-fat from acceptable ingredients)	ketchup, mayonnaise, pickles, pickle relish, Worcestershire sauce
chickweed, coltsfoot, dandelion, dong quai, elder, gentian, goldenseal, hops, horehound, licorice root, linden, mulberry, mullein, parsley, peppermint, rasberry leaf, sage, sarsaparilla, senna, shepherd's purse, skullcap, spearmint, strawberry leaf, thyme, vervain, white birch, white oak bark, yarrow	catnip, cayenne, corn silk, red clover, rhubarb, yellow dock
white wine	beer; distilled liquors; seltzer water; diet cola, cola, and other sodas; black teas (regular & decaf)

Type B Diet

FOOD GROUP *Portion*	FREQUENCY BY ANCESTRAL TYPE	HIGHLY BENEFICIAL
MEAT & **POULTRY:** *portion:* men 4–6 oz. women/ children 2–5 oz.	**WEEKLY** *Lean Red Meats:* Caucasians: 2–3X Africans: 3–4X Asians: 2–3X *Poultry:* Caucasians: 0–3X Africans: 0–2X Asians: 1–2X	lamb, mutton, rabbit, venison
SEAFOOD: *portion:* 4–6 oz.	**WEEKLY** Caucasians: 3–5X Africans: 4–6X Asians: 3–5X	cod, flounder, grouper, haddock, hake, halibut, mackerel, mahimahi, monkfish, ocean perch, pickerel, pike, porgy, sardine, sea trout, shad, sole, sturgeon, sturgeon eggs (caviar)
EGGS & **DAIRY:** *portion:* egg: 1 cheeses: 2 oz. yogurt: 4–6 oz. milk: 4–6 oz.	**WEEKLY** *Eggs:* Caucasians: 3–4X Africans: 3–4X Asians: 5–6X *Cheeses:* Caucasians: 3–5X Africans: 3–4X Asians: 2–3X *Yogurt:* Caucasians: 2–4X Africans: 0–4X Asians: 1–3X *Milk:* Caucasians: 4–5X Africans: 0–3X Asians: 2–3X	cottage cheese, farmer, feta, goat cheese, goat milk, kefir, mozzarella, ricotta, skim or 2% milk, yogurt with fruit, frozen yogurt
OILS & FATS: *portion:* 1 tablespoon	**WEEKLY** Caucasians: 4–6X Africans: 3–5X Asians: 5–7X	olive oil

NEUTRAL	AVOID
beef, ground beef, buffalo, liver, pheasant, turkey, veal	bacon, chicken, Cornish hens, duck, goose, ham, heart, partridge, pork, quail
abalone, albacore (tuna), bluefish, carp, catfish, herring (fresh & pickled), rainbow trout, red snapper, sailfish, salmon, scallop, shark, silver perch, smelt, snapper, squid (calamari), swordfish, tilefish, weakfish, white perch, whitefish, yellow perch	anchovy, barracuda, beluga, bluegill bass, clam, conch, crab, crayfish, eel, frog, lobster, lox (smoked salmon), mussels, octopus, oysters, sea bass, shrimp, snail, striped bass, turtle, yellowtail
Brie, butter, buttermilk, Camembert, casein, Cheddar, Colby, cream cheese, Edam, Emmenthal, Gouda, Gruyère, Jarlsberg, Monterey Jack, Munster, neufchatel, Parmesan, provolone, sherbet, soy cheese, soy milk, Swiss, whey, whole milk	American cheese, blue, ice cream, string cheese
cod liver oil, linseed (flaxseed) oil	canola oil, corn oil, cottonseed oil, peanut oil, safflower oil, sesame oil, sunflower oil

Type B Diet

FOOD GROUP *Portion*	FREQUENCY BY ANCESTRAL TYPE	HIGHLY BENEFICIAL
NUTS & **SEEDS:** *portion:* Nuts & seeds: 6–8 nuts nut butters: 1 tablespoon	**WEEKLY** *Nuts & Seeds:* Caucasians: 2–5X Africans: 3–5X Asians: 2–3X *Nut Butters:* Caucasians: 2–3X Africans: 2–3X Asians: 2–3X	none
BEANS & **LEGUMES:** *portion:* 1 cup dry	**WEEKLY** Caucasians: 2–3X Africans: 3–4X Asians: 4–5X	kidney beans, lima beans, navy beans
CEREALS: *portion:* 1 cup dry	**WEEKLY** Caucasians: 2–4X Africans: 2–3X Asians: 2–4X	millet, oat bran, oatmeal, puffed rice, rice bran, spelt
BREADS & **MUFFINS:** *portion:* 1 slice bread or crackers 1 muffin	**DAILY** All Ancestral Types *Bread/* *Crackers:* 0–1X *Muffins:* 0–1X	brown-rice bread, Essene bread, Ezekiel bread, millet, rice cakes
GRAINS & **PASTA:** *portion:* grains: 1 cup dry pastas: 1 cup dry	**WEEKLY** *Grains:* Caucasians: 3–4X Africans: 3–4X Asians: 2–3X *Pastas:* Caucasians: 3–4X Africans: 3–4X Asians: 2–3X	oat flour, rice flour

NEUTRAL	AVOID
almond butter, almonds, Brazil, chestnuts, hickory, litchis, macadamias, pecans, walnuts	cashews, filberts, pignoli (pine) nuts, pistachio nuts, peanuts, peanut butter, poppy seeds, pumpkin seeds, sesame butter (tahini), sesame seeds, sunflower butter, sunflower seeds
broad beans, cannellini beans, copper beans, fava beans, green beans, jicama beans, northern beans, red beans, snap beans, string beans, tamarind beans, white beans, green peas, pea pods, soy beans	adzuki beans, black beans, garbanzo beans, pinto beans, lentils (domestic, green & red), black-eyed peas
Cream of Rice, Familia, farina, granola, Grape Nuts	amaranth, barley, buckwheat, cornflakes, cornmeal, Cream of Wheat, kamut, rye, seven-grain, shredded wheat, wheat bran, wheat germ
gluten-free bread, high-protein no-wheat bread, oat-bran muffins, spelt bread, soy-flour bread	wheat bagels, corn muffins, durum wheat, multigrain bread, 100% rye bread, rye crisp, Rye Vita, wheat-bran muffins, whole-wheat bread, Fin Crisp, Wasa bread, Ideal flat bread, pumpernickel
graham flour, spelt flour, white flour, semolina pasta, spinach pasta, quinoa, basmati rice, brown rice, white rice	kasha buckwheat, couscous, barley flour, bulgur-wheat flour, durum-wheat flour, gluten flour, rye flour, whole-wheat flour, artichoke pasta, soba noodles, wild rice

Type B Diet

FOOD GROUP *Portion*	FREQUENCY BY ANCESTRAL TYPE	HIGHLY BENEFICIAL

VEGETABLES:
portion:
raw: 1 cup
cooked: 1 cup
          prepared
	DAILY
	All Ancestral
	Types
	Raw:
	          3–5X
	Cooked:
	          3–5X
		beets, beet leaves, broccoli, Chinese cabbage, red cabbage, white cabbage, carrots, cauliflower, collard greens, eggplant, kale, lima beans, shiitake mushrooms, mustard greens, parsley, parsnips, green peppers, jalapeño peppers, red peppers, yellow peppers, sweet potatoes, Brussels sprouts, all types yams

FRUITS:
portion:
     1 fruit or
     3–5 oz.
	DAILY
	All Ancestral
	Types
	          3–4X
		bananas, cranberries, black grapes, concord grapes, green grapes, red grapes, papaya, pineapple, dark plums, green plums, red plums

JUICES &
FLUIDS:
portion: 8 oz.
	DAILY
	All Ancestral
	Types
	Juices:
	          2–3X
	Water:
	          4–7X
		cabbage, cranberry, grape, papaya, pineapple

NEUTRAL	AVOID
arugula, asparagus, bamboo shoots, bok choy, celery, chervil, chicory, cucumber, daikon radish, dandelion, dill, endive, escarole, fennel, fiddlehead ferns, garlic, ginger, horseradish, kohlrabi, leek, bibb lettuce, Boston lettuce, iceberg lettuce, romaine lettuce, mesclun lettuce, abalone mushrooms, domestic mushrooms, enoki mushrooms, Portobello mushrooms, tree oyster mushrooms, okra, green onions, Spanish onions, yellow onions, red potatoes, white potatoes, radicchio, rappini, rutabaga, scallion, seaweed, shallots, snow peas, spinach, alfalfa sprouts, all types squash, Swiss chard, turnips, water chestnuts, watercress, zucchini	domestic & Jerusalem artichoke, avocado, white corn, yellow corn, black olives, green olives, Greek olives, Spanish olives, pumpkin, radishes, mung sprouts, radish sprouts, tempeh, tofu, tomato
apples, apricots, blackberries, blueberries, boysenberries, cherries, black & red currants, dates, elderberries, dried figs, fresh figs, gooseberries, grapefruit, guava, kiwi, kumquat, lemons, limes, loganberries, mangoes, canang melon, cantaloupe, casaba melon, Christmas melon, Crenshaw melon, honeydew melon, musk melon, Spanish melon, watermelon, nectarines, oranges, peaches, pears, plantains, prunes, raisins, raspberries, strawberries, tangerines	coconuts, persimmons, pomegranates, prickly pear, rhubarb, starfruit
apple, apple cider, apricot, carrot, celery, black cherry, cucumber, grapefruit, orange, prune, water with lemon, vegetable juice (corresponding with highlighted vegetables)	tomato

Type B Diet

FOOD GROUP *Portion*	FREQUENCY BY ANCESTRAL TYPE	HIGHLY BENEFICIAL
SPICES:		cayenne pepper, curry, ginger, horse-radish, parsley
CONDIMENTS:		none
HERBAL TEAS:		ginger, ginseng, licorice, licorice root, parsley, peppermint, raspberry leaf, rose hips, sage
MISC. BEVERAGES:		green tea

NEUTRAL	AVOID
agar, anise, arrowroot, basil, bay leaf, bergamot, brown-rice syrup, capers, caraway, cardamom, carob, celery seeds, chervil, chives, chocolate, clove, coriander, cream of tartar, cumin, dill, dulse, garlic, honey, kelp, maple syrup, marjoram, mint, miso, molasses, dry mustard, nutmeg, oregano, paprika, peppercorn pepper, red pepper flakes, peppermint, pimiento, rice syrup, rosemary, saffron, sage, salt, savory, soy sauce, spearmint, white & brown sugar, tamari sauce, tamarind, tarragon, thyme, vanilla extract, apple cider vinegar, balsamic vinegar, red wine vinegar, white vinegar, wintergreen	allspice, almond extract, barley malt, cinnamon, cornstarch, corn syrup, plain gelatin, ground black pepper, white pepper, tapioca
apple butter, jam & jelly from acceptable fruits, mayonnaise, mustard, dill pickles, kosher pickles, sour pickles, sweet pickles, relish, salad dressing (low-fat from acceptable ingredients), Worcestershire sauce	ketchup
alfalfa, burdock, catnip, cayenne, chamomile, chickweed, dandelion, dong quai, echinacea, elder, green tea, hawthorn, horehound, mulberry, St.-John's-wort, sarsaparilla, slippery elm, spearmint, strawberry leaf, thyme, valerian, vervain, white birch, white oak bark, yarrow, yellow dock	aloe, coltsfoot, corn silk, fenugreek, gentian, goldenseal, hops, linden, mullein, red clover, rhubarb, senna, shepherd's purse, skullcap
beer, regular & decaf coffee, black decaf tea, black regular tea, red wine, white wine	distilled liquor, seltzer water, cola, diet cola, other sodas

Type AB Diet

FOOD GROUP *Portion*	FREQUENCY BY ANCESTRAL TYPE	HIGHLY BENEFICIAL
MEAT & **POULTRY:** *portion:* men 4–6 oz. women/ children 2–5 oz.	**WEEKLY** *Lean Red Meats:* Caucasians: 1–3X Africans: 1–3X Asians: 1–3X *Poultry:* Caucasians: 0–2X Africans: 0–2X Asians: 0–2X	lamb, mutton, rabbit, turkey
SEAFOOD: *portion:* 4–6 oz.	**WEEKLY** Caucasians: 3–5X Africans: 3–5X Asians: 4–6X	albacore (tuna), cod, grouper, hake, mackerel, mahimahi, monkfish, ocean perch, pickerel, pike, porgy, rainbow trout, red snapper, sailfish, sardine, sea trout, shad, snail, sturgeon
EGGS & **DAIRY:** *portion:* egg: 1 cheeses: 2 oz. yogurt: 4–6 oz. milk: 4–6 oz.	**WEEKLY** *Eggs:* Caucasians: 3–4X Africans: 3–5X Asians: 2–3X *Cheeses:* Caucasians: 3–4X Africans: 2–3X Asians: 3–4X *Yogurt:* Caucasians: 3–4X Africans: 2–3X Asians: 1–3X *Milk:* Caucasians: 3–6X Africans: 1–6X Asians: 2–5X	cottage cheese, farmer, feta, goat cheese, goat's milk, kefir, mozzarella, ricotta, nonfat sour cream, yogurt
OILS & FATS: *portion:* 1 tablespoon	**WEEKLY** Caucasians: 4–8X Africans: 1–5X Asians: 3–7X	olive oil

NEUTRAL	AVOID
liver, pheasant	bacon, beef, ground beef, buffalo, chicken, Cornish hens, duck, goose, ham, heart, partridge, pork, veal, venison, quail
abalone, bluefish, carp, catfish, caviar, herring (fresh) mussels, salmon, scallop, shark, silver perch, smelt, snapper, squid (calamari), swordfish, tilefish, weakfish, whitefish, white perch, yellow perch	anchovy, barracuda, beluga, bluegill bass, clam, conch, crab, crayfish, eel, flounder, frog, sole, haddock, halibut, herring (pickled), lobster, lox (smoked salmon), octopus, oysters, sea bass, shrimp, striped bass turtle, yellowtail
casein, Cheddar, Colby, cream cheese, Edam, Emmenthal, Gouda, Gruyère, Jarlsberg, Monterey Jack, Munster, neufchatel, skim or 2% milk, soy cheese,* soy milk,* string cheese, Swiss, whey *good dairy alternatives	American cheese, blue, Brie, butter, buttermilk, Camembert, ice cream, Parmesan, provolone, sherbet, whole milk
canola oil, cod liver oil, linseed (flaxseed) oil, peanut oil	corn oil, cottonseed oil, safflower oil, sesame oil, sunflower oil

Type AB Diet

FOOD GROUP *Portion*	FREQUENCY BY ANCESTRAL TYPE	HIGHLY BENEFICIAL
NUTS & **SEEDS:** *portion:* nuts & seeds: 6–8 nuts nut butters: 1 tablespoon	**WEEKLY** *Nuts & Seeds:* Caucasians: 2–5X Africans: 2–5X Asians: 2–3X *Nut Butters:* Caucasians: 3–7X Africans: 3–7X Asians: 2–4X	chestnuts, peanuts, peanut butter, walnuts
BEANS & **LEGUMES:** *portion:* 1 cup dry	**WEEKLY** Caucasians: 2–3X Africans: 3–5X Asians: 4–6X	navy beans, pinto beans, red beans, soy beans, green lentils
CEREALS: *portion:* 1 cup dry	**WEEKLY** Caucasians: 2–3X Africans: 2–3X Asians: 2–4X	millet, oat bran, oatmeal, rice bran, puffed rice, ryeberry, spelt
BREADS & **MUFFINS:** *portion:* 1 slice bread or crackers 1 muffin	**DAILY** All Ancestral Types *Breads/* *Crackers:* 0–1X Muffins: 0–1X	brown-rice bread, Essene bread, Ezekiel bread, Fin crisp, millet, rice cakes, 100% rye bread, rye crisps, Rye Vita, soy-flour bread, sprouted-wheat bread, Wasa bread
GRAINS & **PASTA:** *portion:* grains: 1 cup dry pastas: 1 cup dry	**WEEKLY** *Grains:* Caucasians: 3–4X Africans: 2–4X Asians: 3–4X *Pastas:* Caucasians: 3–4X Africans: 2–3X Asians: 3–4X	oat flour, rice flour, rye flour, sprouted- wheat flour, basmati rice, brown rice, white rice, wild rice

NEUTRAL	AVOID
almond butter, almonds, Brazil, cashew, hickory, litchis, macadamias, pignoli (pine) nuts, pistachios	filberts, poppy seeds, pumpkin seeds, sesame butter (tahini), sesame seeds, sunflower butter, sunflower seeds
broad beans, cannellini beans, copper beans, northern beans, green beans, jicama beans, snap beans, string beans, tamarind beans, white beans, domestic lentils, red lentils, green peas, pods peas	adzuki beans, black beans, fava beans, garbanzo beans, kidney beans, lima beans, black-eyed peas
amaranth, barley, Cream of Rice, Cream of Wheat, Familia, farina, granola, Grape Nuts, seven-grain, shredded wheat, soy flakes, soy granules, wheat bran, wheat germ	buckwheat, corn flakes, cornmeal, kamut
wheat bagels, durum wheat, gluten-free bread, high-protein bread, Ideal flat bread, wheat matzos, multi-grain bread, oat-bran muffins, pumpernickel, spelt bread, wheat bread, wheat-bran muffins, whole-wheat bread	corn muffins
couscous, bulgur wheat flour, durum-wheat flour, gluten flour, graham flour, spelt flour, white flour, whole-wheat flour, semolina pasta, spinach pasta, quinoa	buckwheat, artichoke pasta, soba noodles, barley flour

Type AB Diet

FOOD GROUP Portion	FREQUENCY BY ANCESTRAL TYPE	HIGHLY BENEFICIAL
VEGETABLES: portion: raw, cooked, or steamed: 1 cup prepared	**DAILY** All Ancestral Types *Raw vegetables:* 3–5X *Cooked or steamed:* 3–5X	beet leaves, beets, broccoli, cauliflower, celery, collard greens, cucumber, dandelion, eggplant, garlic, kale, maitake mushrooms, mustard greens, parsley, parsnips, sweet potatoes, alfalfa sprouts, tempeh, tofu, all types yams
FRUITS portion: 1 fruit or 3–5 oz.	**DAILY** All Ancestral Types 3–4X	cherries, cranberries, dried figs, fresh figs, gooseberries, black grapes, concord grapes, green grapes, red grapes, grapefruit, kiwi, lemons, loganberries, pineapples, dark plums, green plums, red plums
JUICES & FLUIDS: portion: 8 oz.	**DAILY** All Ancestral Types *Juices:* 2–3X *Water:* 4–7X	cabbage, carrot, celery, black cherry, cranberry, grape, papaya

NEUTRAL	AVOID
arugula, asparagus, bamboo shoots, bok choy, Chinese cabbage, red cabbage, white cabbage, caraway, carrots, chervil, chicory, coriander, daikon, endive, escarole, fennel, fiddlehead ferns, ginger, horseradish, kohlrabi, leek, bibb lettuce, Boston lettuce, iceberg lettuce, mesclun lettuce, romaine lettuce, abalone mushrooms, domestic mushrooms, portobello mushrooms, tree mushrooms, oyster mushrooms, enoki mushrooms, Shiitake mushrooms, okra, green olives, Greek olives, Spanish olives, green onions, red onions, Spanish onions, yellow onions, red potatoes, white potatoes, pumpkin, radicchio, rappini, rutabaga, scallion, seaweed, shallots, snow peas, spinach, Brussels sprouts, all types squash, Swiss chard, tomato, turnips, water chestnuts, watercress, zucchini	domestic artichokes, Jerusalem artichokes, avocados, white corn, yellow corn, lima beans, black olives, green peppers, jalapeño peppers, red peppers, yellow peppers, radishes, mung sprouts, radish sprouts
apples, apricots, blackberries, blueberries, boysenberries, black & red currants, dates, elderberries, kumquat, limes, canang melon, cantaloupe, casaba melon, Christmas melon, Crenshaw melon, honeydew melon, muskmelon, Spanish melon, watermelon, nectarines, papayas, peaches, pears, plantains, prunes, raisins, raspberries, strawberries, tangerines	bananas, coconuts, guava, mangoes, oranges, persimmons, pomegranates, prickly pears, rhubarb, starfruit (carambola)
apple, apple cider, apricot, cucumber, grapefruit, pineapple, prune, water with lemon, vegetable juice (corresponding with highlighted vegetables)	orange

Type AB Diet

FOOD GROUP *Portion*	FREQUENCY BY ANCESTRAL TYPE	HIGHLY BENEFICIAL
SPICES:		curry, garlic, horseradish, miso, parsley
CONDIMENTS:		none
HERBAL TEAS:		alfalfa, burdock, chamomile, echinacea, ginger, ginseng, green tea, hawthorn, licorice root, rose hips, strawberry leaf
MISC. BEVERAGES:		regular coffee, decaf coffee, green tea

NEUTRAL	AVOID
agar, arrowroot, basil, bay leaf, berg-amot, brown-rice syrup, cardamom, carob, chervil, chive, chocolate, cinna-mon, clove, corriander, cream of tar-tar, cumin, dill, dulse, honey, kelp, maple syrup, marjoram, mint, mo-lasses, dry mustard, nutmeg, paprika, peppermint, rice syrup, rosemary, saf-fron, sage, salt, savory, soy sauce, spearmint, brown sugar, white sugar, tamari, tamarind, tarragon, thyme, turmeric, vanilla, wintergreen, apple cider vinegar, balsamic vinegar, red wine vinegar	allspice, almond extract, anise, barley malt, capers, cornstarch, corn syrup, plain gelatin, ground black pepper, cayenne pepper, peppercorn pepper, red flakes pepper, white pepper, tapi-oca, white vinegar
jam & jelly (from acceptable fruits), mayonnaise, mustard, salad dressing (low-fat from acceptable ingredients)	ketchup, dill pickles, kosher pickles, sweet pickles, sour pickles, relish, Worcestershire sauce
catnip, cayenne, chickweed, dande-lion, dong quai, elder, goldenseal, horehound, mulberry, parsley, pepper-mint, raspberry leaf, sage, St.-John's-wort, sarsaparilla, slippery elm, spearmint, thyme, valerian, vervain, white birch, white oak bark, tarrow, yellow dock	aloe, coltsfoot, corn silk, fenugreek, gentian, hops, linden, mullein, red clover, rhubarb, senna, shepherd's purse, skullcap
beer, seltzer water, club soda, red wine, white wine	distilled liquor, cola soda, diet soda, other soda, black decaf tea, black reg-ular tea

PART II

Recipes

*T*HIS LARGE SELECTION OF RECIPES INCLUDES dishes that are delicious, healthy, imaginative, and right for your blood type. For those who fear that the Blood Type Diet will deprive them of the pure pleasure of eating wonderful foods, these recipes will put their minds at ease. They've been prepared by professional chefs Martine Lloyd Warner and Gabrielle Sindorf. Treat the recipes as suggestions, and invent your own variations.

From time to time, you will come across a box that looks like this:

CYBER RECIPE

Thanks to the wonders of the Web, we've been able to open up the dialogue about the Blood Type Diet to several hundred thousand people. The Recipe Exchange is a popular feature that enables people to share some of their own creations. These recipes have all been certified and tested. They are unique contributions from people just like you who are finding ways to incorporate the diet into their daily lives.

Each recipe is keyed to blood type. Refer to the box at the top of each recipe. Read the key this way:

- HIGHLY BENEFICIAL indicates that the primary ingredients are Highly Beneficial for your type. Minor ingredients may be either Highly Beneficial or Neutral. There are no Avoid ingredients.

- NEUTRAL indicates that the primary ingredients are Neutral for your type. Minor ingredients may be either Neutral or Highly Beneficial. There are no Avoid ingredients.
- AVOID indicates that there are ingredients in the recipe that your type should avoid.

HIGHLY BENEFICIAL		NEUTRAL		AVOID	

The recipes in this section include every food category on your blood type list. There is truly something for everyone.

Contents

Meat & Poultry
Fish & Seafood
Tofu & Tempeh
Pasta
Pizza
Beans & Grains
Vegetables
Soups & Stews
Bread, Muffins, Tea Cakes, & Batters
Salads
Sandwiches, Eggs, Tarts, Frittatas, & Crêpes
Desserts, Cheese, & Fruit
Dressings, Sauces, Chutneys, & Relishes
Beverages
Snacks, Treats, & Munchies

Quick Meals at a Glance

SINCE MOST PEOPLE live in households that include more than one blood type, these recipes provide an easy way to put a meal together without worrying about assembling ingredients for separate meals. When you're in a rush, you can depend on these recipes for a blood type–friendly meal. Post this list on your refrigerator.

Meat & Poultry
turkey burgers
turkey cutlets
roast turkey

Fish & Seafood
Indonesian broiled swordfish
sautéed monkfish
tuna steak marinated in lemon and garlic
steamed whole red snapper

Pasta
broccoli rabe with pasta

Pizza
basic pizza dough
salad pizza
white pizza
zucchini and basil pizza

Beans & Grains
faro pilaf
millet tabbouleh
millet couscous
spelt berry and basmati rice pilaf
quinoa risotto
brown rice pilaf
spelt berry salad

Vegetables
glazed turnips and onions
carrots and parsnips with garlic, ginger, and cilantro
braised fennel with garlic
vegetable fritters
Swiss chard with sardines
braised collards
grilled Portobello mushrooms
sautéed leeks

Soups & Stews
basic turkey stock
basic vegetable stock
turkey soup
gingered squash soup
mixed roots soup
miso soup
hearty fish soup
white bean and wilted greens soup
simple fish soup

Salads
mesclun salad
spinach salad with egg and bacon
Greek salad
carrot-raisin salad
alder-smoked mackerel salad
great Caesar salad
green beans, chèvre, and walnuts

Sandwiches, etc.
grilled goat Cheddar on Ezekiel bread
quick tuna salad
fresh mozzarella, sautéed zucchini, and garlic
soft goat cheese preserves
curried free-range egg salad

grilled cheese on Ezekiel bread
frittata with pasta and carmelized onions
zucchini and mushroom frittata
spinach frittata
crêpes

Desserts
rice-crispy cakes
apple cake
basmati rice pudding
pineapple upside-down cake
sautéed pears or apples
tropical salad
fruit compote or baked apples
apple pie

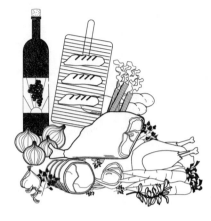

SIX

Meat & Poultry

*T*HE MOST DELICIOUS—AND HEALTHY—WAY TO EAT meat is very lean (trimmed of visible fat), and cooked simply, alone or with vegetables. When you don't have time to cook an elaborate meal, meat is also quick and easy. These recipes include both everyday and special-occasion meals that recapture what we all loved so much about meat and poultry in simpler times.

Try to find an organic source. Most commercially produced meats and poultry are raised on feed that is laced with chemical residues from pesticides, herbicides, and fertilizers. The animals are also fed hormones to increase their rate of growth. There is an enormous effort taking place to produce healthy, relatively pure food, but those efforts need the support of consumers. The greater the demand for organic meat and poultry, the greater the quantity available and the lower the prices.

BEEF BRISKET

HIGHLY BENEFICIAL	O	NEUTRAL	B	AVOID	A, AB

A warming fall and winter dinner. Try adding six yellow onions, the size of your fist, for the last hour of cooking. They add a pleasant savory flavor.

2 tablespoons olive oil
2- to 3-lb. brisket
1 onion, diced
2 cups red wine
4 cloves garlic, crushed and peeled
1 teaspoon dried thyme
3 bay leaves
2 cups boiling water
salt

Heat oil in a heavy casserole pan over low heat. Add brisket and brown on both sides. Add onion and cook several minutes, until golden. Add wine and bring to a boil. Reduce heat and simmer 20 minutes. Add garlic, thyme, bay leaves, and boiling water and bring to a boil again. Reduce heat and simmer 3 hours, turning meat once or twice, until done. Add salt to taste. Brisket needs plenty of time to get tender. *Serves 8.*

CHICKEN OR TURKEY PAPRIKA

HIGHLY BENEFICIAL	AB	NEUTRAL	A, B	AVOID	O

This satisfying recipe is prefect for cooler weather. Type B and Type AB should substitute turkey for the chicken in this recipe.

2 tablespoons olive oil
1 large yellow onion, diced
paprika
1 chicken, cut into 8 pieces
1 to 2 cups water or chicken (turkey) stock
salt
spelt flour
8 oz. sour cream (if too rich, try substituting
some drained yogurt)

Heat oil in a large skillet and sauté onion until golden. Sprinkle paprika liberally over onion and stir to cook paprika; do not scorch. Push onions to side of pan and add chicken. Allow chicken to color on one side, then turn and spoon onions over top of chicken. Allow to color on other side. When chicken parts are a rich red color, add water or stock and bring to a boil. Add salt to taste, reduce heat, and simmer 45 minutes, or until chicken is thoroughly cooked.

Transfer chicken and sauce to a bowl and add 2 to 3 tablespoons flour to the skillet. Slowly pour the liquid from chicken back into the skillet, stirring constantly until thickened. Add sour cream or yogurt and stir. Return chicken or turkey to pan and heat thoroughly. Do not boil. Serve over noodles or rice.
Serves 4 to 8.

ITALIAN CHICKEN

HIGHLY BENEFICIAL		NEUTRAL	O, A	AVOID	B, AB

An uncomplicated chicken dish that is simple to prepare. It lends itself to risotto or pilaf as an accompaniment, and a salad of mixed greens.

3 tablespoons olive oil
1 chicken, cut into 8 pieces

6 to 8 cloves garlic, crushed and peeled
½ teaspoon chopped fresh rosemary
salt
pepper
water or chicken stock

Heat 1 tablespoon oil in a heavy skill over low heat. Add chicken pieces and cook several minutes. When they begin to color, add remaining 2 tablespoons oil and garlic. Turn chicken in the oil. Sprinkle with rosemary, salt, and pepper. Add ½ cup to 1 cup water or stock, and let it come to a boil, then reduce heat and cover skillet. Cook chicken 35 to 45 minutes, checking frequently to make sure there's still liquid in the pan. Add water as needed in small amounts (1 to 2 tablespoons). Chicken will fall away from the bone. Transfer chicken to dinner plates and deglaze the pan with a few tablespoons of water or wine, pouring pan liquid over chicken as sauce.
Serves 4 to 8.

BRAISED RABBIT

HIGHLY BENEFICIAL	B, AB	NEUTRAL	O	AVOID	A

Rabbit has a taste very similar to that of chicken and can be cooked in many of the same ways. This method omits the traditional marinade, necessary for the gamier-tasting hare, resulting in tender, moist meat.

2 tablespoons olive oil
1 rabbit, cut into about 12 pieces
2 tablespoons butter (TYPE AB USE OLIVE OIL)
1 large carrot, diced
4 cloves garlic, chopped
1 stalk celery, finely sliced

1 medium onion, diced
1½ cups white wine
water
salt

Heat oil in a heavy skillet over low heat. Add rabbit pieces and cook until nicely browned. Transfer rabbit to platter. Add butter or olive oil to pan. When melted, add carrot, garlic, celery, and onion, and sauté, turning, until golden. Pushing aside the vegetables, return rabbit to skillet. Spoon vegetables over the pieces and add wine. Cook for a few moments, then add 1 cup water, or enough to braise the rabbit, and bring to a boil. Cover skillet, reduce heat, and check to make sure that there is always enough braising liquid in the pan. Salt to taste. Cook rabbit for at least 90 minutes, or until very tender. Serve with rice. *Serves 3 to 4.*

SIMPLE SESAME CHICKEN

HIGHLY BENEFICIAL		NEUTRAL	O, A	AVOID	B, AB

When you need a good meal but don't have a lot of preparation time, try this simple and delicious recipe. Serve it with rice or spelt noodles and a salad of tossed greens.

8 chicken pieces or breasts on bone
2 tablespoons soy sauce or tamari sauce
3 to 4 cloves garlic, crushed and peeled
¼ cup sesame seeds

Preheat oven to 375 degrees F. Put chicken pieces in a baking dish. Sprinkle each piece with soy sauce. Rub with crushed garlic. Sprinkle sesame seeds over top and bake 50 minutes, or until done. *Serves 4 to 8.*

GRILLED CURRIED LEG OF LAMB

HIGHLY BENEFICIAL	O, B, AB	**NEUTRAL**		**AVOID**	A

Other than the fact that lamb is highly beneficial for three of the four blood types, with the exception of Type A, it has other advantages as well. The meat is tremendously flavorful and also very lean. Even a leg of lamb, once it has been boned and trimmed, is an affordable meat. The serving portions are generous. One leg of lamb can easily serve a family of four for two meals.

This simple but elegant grilled dinner can be made even easier if you grill your vegetables at the same time. Try summer squashes, peppers, eggplant, sweet potatoes, onions . . . whatever your particular Blood Type Diet allows. Use plenty of olive oil and tend closely.

2 tablespoons curry powder
2 tablespoons ground cumin
1 tablespoon salt
2 tablespoons kelp powder
1 tablespoon five-spice powder
1 leg of lamb, boned and butterflied

Combine spices and rub them dry all over leg of lamb. Let sit 1 hour. Prepare grill. Grill lamb 20 minutes on each side for medium rare; 25 to 30 minutes for well done. Remove lamb from grill and let stand 10 minutes, then slice thinly. *Serves 4.*

BROILED LAMB CHOPS

| HIGHLY BENEFICIAL | O, B, AB | NEUTRAL | | AVOID | A |

Lamb chops are very quick and easy to prepare. In fact, the simpler the treatment, the better. Rib chops are fattier and have less meat, but are quite tasty. Loin chops are often smaller, less fatty, and have more meat.

2 to 3 lamb chops per person
1 large clove garlic, peeled and cut
1 tablespoon dry rub of fresh rosemary and salt per serving
olive oil

Preheat broiler. Adjust broiler pan so that the chops are 3 to 4 inches from heat source. Remove excess fat from the chops, and place in a flame-proof pan. Rub meat with cut garlic cloves, then the herb mix. Pour a few teaspoons of olive oil over chops, and turn them once to coat both sides with oil. Place in broiler and cook 5 to 7 minutes on each side, or until meat is well browned. Turn chops and replace under broiler, browning other side as well. Serve with mashed sweet potatoes and braised greens.

TURKEY BURGERS

| HIGHLY BENEFICIAL | AB | NEUTRAL | O, A, B | AVOID | |

Turkey is usually quite lean, so how can it make a good burger? Eggs, onions, and bread add the necessary moisture to make these light and delicious. If you're concerned as to who would eat them, surprise. Children love them!

1 lb. ground turkey
2 slices of spelt or Ezekiel bread
1 tablespoon olive oil
1 medium onion, finely chopped
2 eggs
handful of chopped fresh parsley
pinch of salt
olive oil for frying

Place ground turkey in a large bowl and shred the bread over the meat. In a skillet, heat oil over medium heat. Add onion and sauté until soft and golden; add to bowl. Beat eggs in a small bowl until light and pour into bowl with turkey. Add chopped parsley and salt. With your hands, mix the ingredients gently but completely, using a very light touch. Do not condense the mixture; keep it fluffy. When ingredients are well mixed, shape them into 5 or 6 patties and cook in olive oil over medium heat until brown, about 5 minutes. Turn and continue to cook another 5 minutes. Cover pan, reduce heat, and let them steam just a little, until the juices run clear. This also keeps the turkey burgers moist. *Serves 5 to 6.*

GRILLED LOIN LAMB CHOPS

HIGHLY BENEFICIAL	O, B, AB	NEUTRAL		AVOID	A

These grilled chops are an easy outdoor meal. The marinade would also work for a butterflied leg of lamb.

6 to 8 double-loin chops or 1 leg of lamb, butterflied
Tamari-Mustard Marinade

Marinate lamb in tamari-mustard marinade 1 to 2 hours. Prepare grill. Grill lamb over medium heat 15 minutes on each side for chops, or 30 to 35 minutes on each side for boneless leg. Let sit 10 minutes before serving.   *Serves 6 to 8.*

TAMARI-MUSTARD MARINADE

Brush this on chicken parts before you grill them or bake them in the oven. It is also very good on tuna steaks.

¼ cup tamari sauce
2 tablespoons Dijon mustard or dry mustard
1 tablespoon honey
2 cloves garlic, minced
zest and juice of 1 lemon
1 tablespoon ground ginger
1 tablespoon ground cumin
2 tablespoons olive oil (TYPE O MAY USE SESAME OIL, IF DESIRED)

Mix all ingredients together and store, tightly covered, in refrigerator.   *Makes about ¾ cup marinade.*

CHICKEN OREGANO

HIGHLY BENEFICIAL		NEUTRAL	O, A	AVOID	B, AB

A perfect dinner when you're in a rush. It's also ideal "picnic" chicken, served warm or cold.

1 cup spelt bread crumbs made from heels of bread
¼ cup grated pecorino romano
3 tablespoons dried oregano or ¼ cup chopped fresh
2 tablespoons kelp powder
8 chicken pieces or breasts on bone

Preheat oven to 375 degrees F. Combine all ingredients, except chicken. Roll each piece of chicken in the seasoning mix. Put pieces in baking dish and bake 50 minutes or until done. *Serves 4 to 8.*

PEANUT OR ALMOND CHICKEN

HIGHLY BENEFICIAL		NEUTRAL	O, A	AVOID	B, AB

This is a delectable cold chicken dish that can serve either as an entrée or an hors d'oeuvre. Type O should use almonds, and Type A, peanuts.

2 lbs. boneless chicken breasts
2 cups unsalted, dry-roasted peanuts or almonds
Pineapple Chutney-Yogurt Sauce (see page 329)
shredded lettuce (optional)

Poach, then cool and drain the chicken breasts. Cut into finger-length pieces; set aside. Toast nuts by placing them in a skillet over medium heat and stirring them around for a few minutes. Watch carefully to make sure they don't scorch. When cool, place nuts in the bowl of a food processor or in a blender, and pulse until they are finely chopped. Dip the chicken in the mayonnaise, then roll each piece in the nuts. Carefully arrange on a serving tray or on a bed of lettuce. *Serves 6 to 8.*

OLD-FASHIONED YANKEE POT ROAST

HIGHLY BENEFICIAL	O	NEUTRAL	B	AVOID	A, AB

This is the kind of dinner to prepare when you'll be home for a good part of the day. Long, slow simmering is the best method for cooking this particular cut of meat. This is also a good dish to make a day ahead, refrigerate overnight, and serve the following night. Once the pot has had a chance to chill, the fat hardens and can easily be skimmed off. Prepare some spelt noodles and serve with the pot roast for a great, comforting meal on a chilly fall or winter night.

There's a choice of stock for this recipe, but please avoid bouillon cubes with MSG. Read the labels. If you need to use water, that's okay; just add more vegetables to the pot: zucchini or other squash, leeks, and garlic. By using water and the extra vegetables, you're making the stock as you go.

¼ cup canola or olive oil for browning
3- to 4-lb. chuck roast from the shoulder
4 cups stock (chicken, beef, or vegetable) or water
1 sprig each fresh rosemary, marjoram, thyme
1 bay leaf
2 large carrots
2 stalks celery
1 large onion
1 sweet potato

In a large pot, heat oil over medium to high heat for 1 minute. Add meat and brown on both sides. Add the stock, herbs and salt, and bring to a boil. Reduce heat and simmer 1 to 1½ hours. Peel and cut vegetables into smaller pieces, and add to the pot. Cook another 45 to 60 minutes. Check meat for tenderness. If necessary, continue to cook an additional 20 to 30 minutes, or until done. Drain off pan juices before serving. *Serves 4 to 6—and makes great leftovers.*

GREAT MEAT LOAF

HIGHLY BENEFICIAL	O	NEUTRAL		AVOID	A, B, AB

The key to a light and fluffy meat loaf depends on the quality of the ingredients and a minimum of handling. This recipe is a protein-packed main course, which, leftover, makes great sandwiches.

1 egg
1 cup soy milk or chicken stock
3 slices of stale bread (Ezekiel or spelt)
1 lb. ground organic beef
1 lb. ground free-range turkey
2 tablespoons kelp powder
1 tablespoon ground cumin
2 tablespoons tamari sauce
3 tablespoons tomato paste

In a large bowl, beat egg and mix in the soy milk or chicken stock. Cut stale bread into cubes and soak in egg and milk mixture until soggy. Add remaining ingredients and mix together in the bowl. Preheat oven to 375 degrees F. Form meat into a 10 × 5 × 5-inch loaf, and bake on a sheet pan 1 hour and 15 minutes, or until juices run clear. Let sit 10 minutes before serving. Cut into 1-inch-thick slices and serve with spelt noodles. *Serves 4.*

SKEWERED LAMB KABOBS

HIGHLY BENEFICIAL	O, B, AB	NEUTRAL		AVOID	A

Lamb is so delicious marinated and then grilled on an open fire. This recipe is a good way to make use of the other half of the leg of lamb used in Indian Lamb Stew with Spinach, page 226.

2 lbs. lamb cubes, cut from the leg
Tamari-Lime Marinade (see next page)

Combine lamb and marinade and leave in the refrigerator anywhere from a couple of hours to a couple of days. When you're ready to grill, choose from the following list of vegetables:

TYPES O AND B

2 red peppers, cut into 2-inch squares
1 large onion, quartered
1 zucchini, cut into 1-inch-thick slices

TYPE AB

1 eggplant, cut into 2-inch squares
1 large onion, quartered
12 mushrooms, left whole

Prepare grill. On long stainless-steel skewers, alternate vegetables and lamb, using about 4 pieces of meat per skewer. The more vegetables, the better. Grill over medium to high heat about 20 minutes, turning frequently. Serve over rice or with spelt pita. For Type B and Type AB, serve the shish kabob with either Cucumber-Yogurt Sauce, page 328, or Pineapple Chutney-Yogurt Sauce, page 329. *Serves 4.*

TAMARI-LIME MARINADE

3 tablespoons Garlic-Shallot Mixture (see page 334)
¼ cup olive oil
2 tablespoons tamari sauce
juice of 1 lime
1 tablespoon ground cumin

Mix all ingredients together. This marinade can be used by every blood type.

TURKEY CUTLETS

HIGHLY BENEFICIAL	AB	NEUTRAL	O, A, B	AVOID	

A nice change from a large roast is the presliced turkey breast meat than can be cooked in a matter of minutes. This is a good choice for a small family or for singles on a night when time is short. Leftover cutlets also make quick and easy sandwiches.

2 tablespoons olive oil
1 package turkey cutlets (about 1 pound)
¼ cup spelt bread crumbs
squeeze of lemon juice
salt

In a large skillet, heat oil over medium-high heat until very hot but not smoking. Dredge each cutlet in bread crumbs and slip into pan, being careful not to overcrowd. Do two batches if necessary. Cook 4 to 5 minutes on each side or until nicely browned, turning once only. Serve with a squeeze of lemon. Salt to taste. *Serves 4.*

LIVER AND ONIONS

HIGHLY BENEFICIAL	O	NEUTRAL	B, AB	AVOID	A

Perfectly cooked liver is a true joy, contrary to our old images from childhood. There are many kinds of liver: beef liver, calf's liver, chicken liver, and lamb liver. Cod, skate, and monkfish livers are also prized. Liver is the body's cleansing station, filtering impurities from the blood, so many toxins are liable to be concentrated in it. Strict regulations are in place so that liver is safe for human consumption. It is also a nutritional powerhouse, rich in iron, protein, and other vitamins and minerals. The best and safest way to eat liver is to find a fresh and organic source. Frozen organic is also widely available.

2 tablespoons plus ¼ cup clarified butter or light olive oil,
according to type
1 large onion, peeled and thinly sliced
3 tablespoons Madeira or sherry
1 lb. sliced liver (whatever is available organically)
½ cup spelt flour (¼ white and ¼ whole is fine)
salt

In a medium skillet, heat 2 tablespoons of the butter or oil. Add onion and cook until wilted and slightly browned. Add Madeira, cook 1 more minute, and set aside.

In a large skillet, heat the remaining butter or oil at medim heat until very hot, but not smoking. Meanwhile, dredge the liver in the flour, 1 piece at a time, shaking off any excess flour, and cook 4 to 5 minutes on each side, turning once only. Be careful not to overcrowd the pan. Salt to taste. Serve liver smothered with onion. *Serves 4 to 5.*

FLANK STEAK

HIGHLY BENEFICIAL	O	NEUTRAL	B	AVOID	A, AB

Flank steak is a surprisingly lean cut of beef that really tastes best cooked on the grill. It also broils very nicely and takes almost no time, depending on its thickness. About ten minutes on each side usually produces a medium-rare to medium piece of meat. Be sure to slice it super thin and on an angle for a flavorful and tender steak.

> *2 tablespoons minced garlic*
> *2 tablespoons ground cumin*
> *1 tablespoon ground cayenne powder*
> *1 tablespoon ground coriander*
> *½ teaspoon ground cloves*
> *½ teaspoon red pepper flakes*
> *1 tablespoon salt*
> *1- to 1½-lb. flank steak*

Prepare grill. Mix the garlic, spices, and salt together and rub generously over the flank steak. Grill meat over medium fire 8 to 10 minutes on each side. Allow to rest 5 minutes before slicing. Serve with Fresh Mint Sauce (see page 332) as a refreshing contrast to the spicy rub.   *Serves 4 to 6.*

ROAST TURKEY

HIGHLY BENEFICIAL	AB	NEUTRAL	O, A, B	AVOID	

There's always a good reason to roast a small turkey or breast of turkey. It no longer has to be reserved for a holiday or company meal. Roasting a turkey is a smart way to prepare for the upcoming week of meals. Of course, that doesn't mean you have to eat turkey for breakfast, lunch, and dinner. Serve dinner the first evening, then slice breast meat for sandwiches the next day. Make a turkey pot pie a little later in the week, and then freeze the carcass until the following weekend and make stock. From there, make a soup!

8 to 12-lb. turkey or 2½- to 3½-lb. turkey breast on the bone
fresh sage or rosemary
1 tablespoon salt

There are no secrets to roasting a great turkey. It's not even necessary to season it, stuff it, truss it, or time it. The pop-up timers that most birds come with now are a great help, even though it's best to cook the birds a few minutes longer. The rule is 15 to 18 minutes per pound, or until the juices run clear when the bird is poked in the thigh. A 10-pound turkey will roast for a good 2½ hours. Always allow the roasted bird to rest 10 minutes before carving. This allows the meat and juices time to settle, and makes it easier to slice.

Preheat oven to 375 degrees F. Remove all giblets and any other innards from the turkey, front and back. Save them for a future stock by freezing in a Zip-loc bag. Rinse the cavity, pat dry with paper towels, and rub the bird with the herbs and salt. If that is unappealing to you, then place the herbs in the cavity and sprinkle with salt. Roast in the preheated oven until done. If the bird is large, you can make a tent out of foil to cover the breast for the first 1½ hours, but don't forget to remove the foil for the last hour of cooking. Crispy brown skin is part of the whole appeal. When finished, please be careful removing the hot roasting pan from the oven. Make sure the surface on which you place the turkey is close by.

🍴 C Y B E R   R E C I P E 🍴

VENISON MEATBALLS WITH MISO GRAVY

AUTHOR: Micayla (sacredworld@yahoo.com)

TYPE O, B

This is a recipe I concocted one day with venison that was given to me from a family member and whatever else I had on hand. Os can do this if they omit the cheese, which will affect the flavor a bit.

MEATBALLS

½ pound ground venison
¼ cup grated romano cheese
2 tablespoons chopped cilantro
1 egg, beaten
1 small onion, finely chopped
2 cloves garlic, finely chopped
1 tablespoon olive oil

GRAVY

2 cups water
1 tablespoon wheat-free tamari sauce
1 tablespoon arrowroot powder mixed with ½ cup water
2 tablespoons white miso

Mix together all meatball ingredients, except oil, and form into little balls. Heat oil in skillet over medium heat. Add meatballs and sauté 20 minutes. Add water and tamari, and cook 30 minutes more.

Combine arrowroot powder with water; add to meatballs and cook until broth thickens slightly. Scoop out ½ cup of broth and add miso, mixing well. Return mixture to meatballs but do not boil. Adjust seasonings.

Makes 4 to 6 servings.

ROAST CHICKEN WITH GARLIC AND HERBS

HIGHLY BENEFICIAL		NEUTRAL	O, A	AVOID	B, AB

A roast chicken can make a good meal any night of the week, and garlic is good for everyone. This simple dish takes only a few minutes to prepare.

1 large chicken
10 cloves garlic, crushed and peeled
2 tablespoons herbes de Provence *(or use rosemary,*
thyme, marjoram, and oregano)
1 teaspoon salt

Preheat oven to 375 degrees F. Prepare the chicken for baking, and rub well with a little of the garlic. Place remaining garlic in the cavity and season the chicken with the herbs and salt. Bake 1 hour and 15 minutes, or until juices run clear. Allow to rest 5 to 10 minutes before carving.   *Serves 4 to 6.*

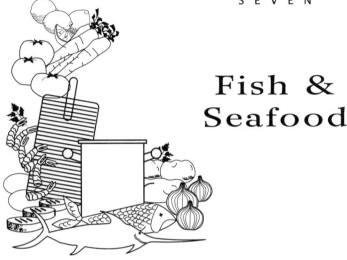

Fish & Seafood

VERY BLOOD TYPE CAN SAMPLE THE WONDERS OF the rivers, lakes, and sea. Seafood, by which we mean crustaceans, such as shrimp and lobster; and mollusks, such as scallops, clams, and oysters, is a little trickier. While all fish and seafood are rich sources of protein and other nutrients, they are blood type–specific. Check your lists.

Many fish run seasonally, and they are much better eating when you buy them at the height of their availability. Imported fish generally has been frozen, and so differs markedly in texture from fresh fish. Fish also harbor parasites, some species more than others. Always cook fish thoroughly.

Short, simple cooking procedures seem to bring out the best qualities in fish. Overcooking makes it tough and dry. Fish can lose its delicate freshness and nutritional benefits very quickly.

SHRIMP KABOBS

HIGHLY BENEFICIAL		NEUTRAL	O	AVOID	A, B, AB

juice of 1 lemon
¼ cup olive oil
3 cloves garlic, crushed and peeled
2 tablespoons chopped fresh parsley
1 stalk lemongrass, bottom third only, peeled and chopped
1-inch piece fresh ginger, peeled and chopped or grated
1 lb. large shrimp, cleaned and deveined

Combine all ingredients, except shrimp, in a medium bowl. Add
the shrimp and marinate, turning to coat thoroughly, at least 4
hours. The longer you marinate the better. Overnight would
be best.

Prepare grill. Place 4 to 6 shrimp on each skewer and grill over
high heat 3 minutes on each side.   *Serves 2.*

BROILED SALMON WITH LEMONGRASS

HIGHLY BENEFICIAL	O, A	NEUTRAL	AB	AVOID	B

3 stalks lemongrass, bottom third only, finely chopped
3 tablespoons soy sauce
2 tablespoons peeled and coarsely grated ginger
2 plum tomatoes (TYPE O ONLY)
2 tablespoons fresh cilantro, chopped finely
juice of 1 lemon
2 scallions, thinly sliced
4 to 6 salmon fillets or steaks, 1 to 1½ pounds

Combine all ingredients, except salmon. Put salmon on large platter and pour marinade over the whole fillet. Let marinate approximately 2 hours.

Preheat broiler. Remove salmon from marinade and broil 15 minutes for medium, 20 minutes for well done.   *Serves 4 to 6.*

SAUTÉED GROUPER

HIGHLY BENEFICIAL	A, B, AB	NEUTRAL	O	AVOID	

This is a fish dish that will delight the kids. It's easy and beats frozen fish sticks by a country mile.

3 tablespoons olive oil
1- to 1½-lb. fresh grouper, trimmed of bones
and cut into finger-sized pieces
¼ cup quinoa flour
salt

In a large cast-iron skillet, heat oil over medium heat. Roll grouper in the flour, shaking off excess. Slip each piece into the hot oil, being careful not to overcrowd the pan. Cook in small batches, adding more oil to the pan if necessary. Make sure the oil is very hot before adding the fish. Turn once when nicely browned on one side, then cook another 3 to 4 minutes. Test for doneness. Pat off excess oil on a paper towel and serve. *Serves 3 to 4.*

SWORDFISH WITH CHERRY TOMATOES, RED ONION, AND BASIL

HIGHLY BENEFICIAL	O	NEUTRAL	AB	AVOID	A, B

This is a colorful and moist swordfish dish. You can use the same preparation for halibut, mako shark, and any other dense, steak-like fish.

2 tablespoons olive oil
2 cloves garlic crushed and peeled
1 lb. swordfish
water
1 small red onion, chopped
1 cup yellow or red cherry tomatoes, halved
½ cup fresh basil, chopped
splash of white wine (optional)

Heat oil over low heat. Add garlic and sauté gently. Add swordfish, distributing the garlic around it. Add ½ cup water. Cover pan and steam swordfish 7 to 10 minutes. Turn fish and steam another 2 to 3 minutes. Add onion and halved tomatoes. Steam 5 more minutes. The onion and tomatoes should be soft. Add basil and cook another moment. Arrange the swordfish and all the vegetables on a plate, using the vegetables as a sauce for the fish. If desired, deglaze pan with a splash of wine, pour over fish, and serve.   *Serves 2.*

INDONESIAN BROILED SWORDFISH

HIGHLY BENEFICIAL	O	NEUTRAL	A, B, AB	AVOID	

This is an easy Asian-inspired dish. Serve it with steamed rice and a fruit salad for a light, healthful meal.

3 tablespoons tamari sauce
2 cloves garlic, minced
2 tablespoons olive oil
1 tablespoon honey
1 tablespoon tahini (ground sesame seeds)
juice of 1 lemon
1 tablespoon ground cumin
1 tablespoon chopped fresh cilantro
2 lbs. swordfish

TYPE B: Replace tahini with 1 tablespoon almond butter.

TYPE AB: Replace tahini with 1 tablespoon peanut butter or almond butter.

Combine all ingredients, except swordfish. Put swordfish on large platter and pour marinade over it. Turn fish once. Allow to marinate at least 1 hour. Turn again.

Preheat broiler and place fish as close to heat source as possible. Broil 5 to 8 minutes on each side, depending on the thickness of the steak. Make sure the interior of the fish is properly cooked. *Serves 4.*

PETER'S SNAILS

HIGHLY BENEFICIAL	A, AB	NEUTRAL	O	AVOID	B

Most snail—or escargot—recipes rely on lots of butter and garlic. You never have a chance to taste the real flavor of the snails. It's an experience not to be duplicated. This is a favorite recipe among the Type As in the D'Adamo household. You can even use canned snails. Since snails have tremendous healing properties for As and ABs, make this simple dish a regular part of your diet.

¼ cup olive oil
2 tablespoons garlic, peeled, chopped, and pressed
12 escargot
parsley flakes

Preheat broiler. Combine oil and garlic in a small bowl and mash into a paste using back of spoon. Arrange escargot on a broiling sheet and brush them with garlic paste. Broil about 10 minutes. When they're almost done, sprinkle them with fresh parsley flakes and broil another minute.   *Serves 2.*

BROILED SALMON STEAKS

HIGHLY BENEFICIAL	O, A	NEUTRAL	B, AB	AVOID	

This is quick and easy for a mixed–blood type family.

4 salmon steaks
1 tablespoon Garlic-Shallot Mixture (see page 334)
2 tablespoons olive oil
juice of 1 lemon

salt
3 tablespoons chopped fresh dill (optional)
lemon wedges (optional)

Preheat broiler. Rub steaks with Garlic-Shallot Mixture, oil, lemon, and salt. Cook fish as close to heat source as possible about 4 to 8 minutes on each side. Test for doneness by prodding with a fork to see if the flesh separates easily. Salmon steaks can be served hot or cold, and dressed with fresh chopped dill and a wedge or two of lemon.   *Serves 4.*

SAUTÉED MONKFISH

HIGHLY BENEFICIAL	A, B, AB	NEUTRAL	O	AVOID	

Monkfish is an excellent fish to cut into chunks and dredge in flour for sautéeing. It can also be used for grilled kabobs on a skewer. Monkfish is often referred to as the poor man's lobster. When cooked, its taste and texture is said to resemble that of the prized crustacean.

1½ lb. monkfish
3 tablespoons olive oil
1 teaspoon dried oregano
brown rice or spelt flour
1 to 2 eggs
salt

Cut the monkfish into 1-inch cubes. Heat oil in a heavy cast-iron skillet over medium heat. Combine oregano and flour. Beat the eggs well. Dip the monkfish pieces in the egg, a few pieces at a time, then roll them in the seasoned flour. Slide floured fish into skillet, but do not overcrowd the pan. Sauté gently, several minutes on each side, until batter is crisp and fish is done. Season with salt.   *Serves 4.*

TUNA STEAK MARINATED IN LEMON AND GARLIC

HIGHLY BENEFICIAL	AB	NEUTRAL	O, A, B	AVOID	

Tuna is certainly a popular fish, though most people are more familiar with canned tuna fish than with any other kind. Maybe this simple but elegant recipe will help to change that.

Serve this tuna with basmati rice, using the cooked marinade as a light sauce over the rice.

1-lb. tuna steak
2 to 3 tablespoons olive oil
juice of 1 lemon
3-inch piece lemon peel
4 cloves garlic, crushed and peeled
2 tablespoons fresh cilantro, chopped
1-inch piece fresh ginger, grated
1 to 2 tablespoons tamari sauce
water

Place tuna in glass or ceramic bowl. Combine oil, lemon juice, lemon peel, garlic, cilantro, ginger, and tamari and pour over fish. Allow to marinate 2 hours, turning a couple of times.

Heat a heavy cast-iron skillet over medium heat. Put tuna in the skillet. Add marinade and a tablespoon or two of water and bring to a simmer. Cover and steam 8 to 10 minutes. Watch carefully; cooking time will vary according to the thickness of the fish and your preference. Add additional water, 1 tablespoon at time, if necessary. *Serves 4.*

STEAMED WHOLE RED SNAPPER

HIGHLY BENEFICIAL	O, AB	NEUTRAL	A, B	AVOID	

Any small, whole, white-fleshed fish can be steamed by this method. Varying the sauce permits you a wide range of possibilities! (See "Dressings, Sauces, Chutneys, & Relishes.") Steam fish on a heavy, restaurant-style platter that fits inside the top of a steaming utensil. A large wok, bamboo steamer, or a traditional fish poacher with removable colander tray modified to lift fish above the boiling water are all suitable alternatives. It is worth working out some kind of system for this recipe because not only is it easy, it provides a meal for all blood types, using their personalized sauces.

*1½- to 2-lb. red snapper, head and tail on, washed,
cleaned, scaled, and trimmed
3 tablespoon olive oil
3 cloves garlic
5 scallions, thinly sliced
1-inch piece fresh ginger, slivered
2 tablespoons tamari sauce
1 scallion, slivered lengthwise
½ cup chopped fresh cilantro*

Steam fish 10 to 15 minutes. Meanwhile, prepare sauce: Heat oil in heavy cast-iron skillet over low to medium heat. Add garlic, scallions, and ginger and gently sauté until softened but not browned. Remove pan from heat and add tamari. When fish is done, drain off accumulated juices and pour sauce over fish. Garnish with slivered scallion and cilantro. *Serves 3 to 4.*

BLUEFISH WITH GARLIC AND PARSLEY

| HIGHLY BENEFICIAL | O | NEUTRAL | B, AB | AVOID | A |

Bluefish is a rich fish, but there is nothing tastier than a really fresh bluefish sizzling on a summer grill. An ocean fish, blues are rich in beneficial oils for Types O, B, and AB. Like mackerel and other fish high in omega-3 oils, the strong taste takes some getting used to, but the result is rewarding.

3 tablespoons olive oil
1 to 1½ lbs. bluefish
4 cloves garlic, crushed and peeled
pinch of salt
½ handful fresh parsley, chopped

Preheat oven to 350 degrees F or use a hot grill. Oil a heavy, oven-proof skillet with 1 tablespoon oil and place fillets skin side down. Pour remaining 2 tablespoons olive oil over the top of the fillets; scatter garlic and a little salt. Bake 10 to 15 minutes, or until done. Sprinkle with chopped parsley.
Serves 4 to 6.

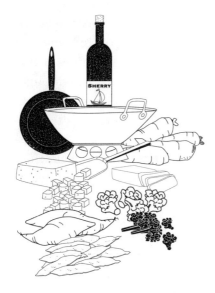

Tofu &
Tempeh

OFU IS THE JAPANESE NAME FOR THE CURD PRODUCED from the milklike liquid extracted from the soybean. It originated in China, where it was known as *doufu*. The soybean is one of the five sacred grains of China, and tofu is a staple throughout Asia. It is the primary source of protein for millions of people. Tofu's texture ranges from soft to firm to extra firm. The silken tofu, however, is soft, delicate, and custardy. Tofu is eaten in countless ways, its bland taste making it perfect for flavorful sauces, spices, and seasonings and its texture lending itself to almost any cooking method.

In particular, Blood Types A and AB should experiment with tofu. Try using it in soups and stews, in place of meat or chicken. It is very inexpensive, easy to find, lasts for several days in the refrigerator, and can be served at any meal.

Tempeh has been a food staple in Indonesia for over two

thousand years. It can be found today in many supermarkets and health-food stores in the refrigerated section. Tempeh is a fermented and pressed rectangular cake composed of soybeans and a fermenting culture called *Rhizopus oligosporus*. This is a filamentous fungus that produces a white mold that spreads throughout the tempeh cake. The tempeh texture alters, and the mold forms a sort of cheeselike rind around its outside. The tempeh becomes extremely nutty and chewy, with a dense, almost meatlike consistency. Some people compare it to a nutty veal. Tempeh can also be made with rice, quinoa, peanuts, kidney beans, wheat, oats, barley, or coconut. It is very popular in vegetarian cuisine worldwide.

Tempeh is substantial, satisfying, and versatile. Great on the grill, fried, baked, or sautéd, tempeh is a perfect protein. It can last unopened in the refrigerator for a couple of weeks, but once opened it should be cooked within a few days. Tempeh should be steamed whole before additional cooking, but if it's left to marinate long enough, the steam step can be eliminated. Black spots on the surface are normal, but if tempeh turns color or smells sour, it should be discarded.

TOFU AND CURRIED VEGETABLE STEW

HIGHLY BENEFICIAL	A, AB	NEUTRAL	O	AVOID	B

Curried vegetables are easy to prepare, and when combined with tofu and brown rice, they form the base for a high protein meal. Choose the most suitable vegetables for your stew, and adjust proportions to balance flavors. The stew may seem a bit thin, but if you include white potato or okra, they will thicken the broth.

2 tablespoons olive oil
4 cloves garlic, chopped
1 medium onion, diced

1 to 2 tablespoons curry powder
2 cups water
2 small turnips, halved and thinly sliced
1 small sugar pumpkin, cut into 1-inch cubes
1 small winter squash, cut into 1-inch pieces
1 carrot, thinly sliced
1 parsnip, thinly sliced
1 white potato, diced (TYPE AB)
1 sweet potato, diced (TYPES O, AB)
½ head cauliflower, cut into "flowers" (TYPES A, AB)
½ head broccoli, cut into "flowers"
12 okra, stemmed and left whole
1 large cake tofu, cubed
½ cup cilantro, chopped

Heat oil in a large, heavy skillet over medium heat. Add garlic and onion and cook, stirring, until just colored. Sprinkle curry powder to taste over vegetables in pan, and continue to gently sauté everything about 5 minutes, being careful not to scorch the garlic and curry. Add water and bring to a boil. Begin adding ingredients, starting with those that require the longest cooking times. When the water has returned to a boil, cover, lower heat, and simmer about 15 minutes, or until all the vegetables are nearly tender. The cauliflower, broccoli, and okra should be put in at this time, and the stew simmered another 10 to 15 minutes or so. Add the tofu for the final 5 minutes, just to heat it through. Ladle over bowls of brown rice and top with a little cilantro. *Serves 6 to 8.*

TOFU-VEGETABLE STIR-FRY

HIGHLY BENEFICIAL	A, AB	NEUTRAL	O	AVOID	B

Stir-fry meals always seem quick, with surprisingly little clean-up. By the time the brown rice is cooked, which takes about forty-five minutes, you'll have had plenty of time to prepare and cut up the rest of the ingredients. Once you begin to stir-fry, the meal will be ready and on the table in a little over 10 minutes.

2 tablespoons olive oil
1 medium onion, diced
1 head broccoli, cut into "flowers," stems sliced
1 small bunch bok choy, cut into 1-inch pieces
6 cloves garlic, crushed and peeled
½ cup vegetable stock or water
½ lb. snow peas
1 cake tofu, cut into ½-inch cubes
1 tablespoon tamari sauce
arrowroot flour (optional)

In a wok or a large, heavy skillet, heat oil over fairly high heat. Add onion, stirring constantly, until the onions are soft. Add broccoli, stirring a moment or two. Add bok choy, stirring again. Add garlic. Add about ½ cup vegetable stock or water and let come to a boil. Cover pan and reduce heat and steam vegetables several minutes, until broccoli is tender but still crisp. Add snow peas, then tofu. Reduce heat and let the mixture steam a few minutes. Add tamari, toss gently, and serve. If you prefer a thick sauce, push the vegetables to one side, add a teaspoon or so of arrowroot flour to the liquid, and stir until thickened. Gently toss with the vegetables before serving. *Serves 4 to 6.*

🍴 CYBER RECIPE 🍴

TASTY TOFU-PUMPKIN STIR-FRY

THE AUTHOR: Ruby (arubastar@foxinternet.net)

TYPE A, AB

This dish gives you that comfort-food feeling and makes your kitchen smell wonderful!

One small sugar-pie pumpkin, diced (raw)
oil
1 package honey sesame–flavored baked tofu, diced
(or flavor of your choice)
about ¼ teaspoon cinnamon
about ¼ teaspoon nutmeg
about ⅛ teaspoon cloves
steamed brown rice
salt (optional)

While the rice is steaming, stir-fry diced pumpkin in oil of your choice. (I used sunflower because I like the nutty flavor it adds.) When pumpkin begins to soften, add spices and stir-fry a minute or so. Add diced tofu and stir-fry until tofu if heated through. Serve stir-fried mixture over rice. Add salt if desired. *Makes 2 to 3 servings.*

TOFU-SESAME FRY

HIGHLY BENEFICIAL	A, AB	NEUTRAL	O	AVOID	B

Tofu can make a satisfying breakfast when served with some brown rice and miso, a deeply complex and salty paste made from fermented soybeans.

2 tablespoons olive oil
1 cake tofu
1 to 2 tablespoons white sesame seeds (TYPE A AND O)
1 to 2 tablespoons black sesame seeds (TYPE A AND O)
2 to 4 tablespoons peanuts, coarsely chopped (TYPE AB)
salt
lemon juice
3 to 4 tablespoons tahini (TYPE A AND O)
juice of ½ lemon (optional)
1 teaspoon tamari sauce (optional)

Heat oil in a heavy skillet over medium to high heat. Slice tofu about ½ inch thick. Coat half the slices with the white seeds, the other half with the black, or coat slices with chopped peanuts. Carefully sauté tofu in the oil, a few minutes on each side. Serve with a dash of salt and a squeeze of lemon. Or drizzle a little tahini, thinned with a little lemon juice and 1 teaspoon tamari, over the tofu. Allow 2 slices per serving. *Serves 3 to 4.*

QUINOA TEMPEH WITH RICE NOODLES

HIGHLY BENEFICIAL	A, AB	NEUTRAL	O	AVOID	B

1 package tempeh (any variety)
2 tablespoons olive oil

1 onion, thinly sliced
2 cloves garlic, crushed and peeled
3 tablespoons chopped fresh cilantro
2 Portobello mushrooms
¼ cup dry cooking sherry
1 package fresh spinach, cleaned and chopped
1 tablespoon tamari sauce
1 lb. rice noodles

Bring a large pot of water to a boil. Boil tempeh 5 to 10 minutes. With a large slotted spoon or strainer, lift tempeh out of boiling water, reserving the water for the noodles; set tempeh aside. In a large skillet, heat oil over medium to high heat. Add onion, garlic, cilantro, and mushrooms and sauté. Slice the tempeh and add the onion and mushroom mixture. Add the sherry, the spinach, and the tamari. Cover and simmer 15 minutes. Meanwhile, cook noodles according to directions and drain. Divide noodles among 4 plates and serve each with 2 slices of tempeh and vegetables. *Serves 4.*

RICE STICKS AND TOFU WITH VEGETABLES

HIGHLY BENEFICIAL	A, AB	NEUTRAL	O	AVOID	B

These rice sticks are not the same as the rice spaghetti you find in the stores. They are, instead, similar in texture to bean threads. Of course, many vegetables are wonderful to use in this dish, so feel free to experiment with what is available in the market or your refrigerator.

MARINADE

½ cup tamari sauce
⅓ cup rice wine

1 tablespoon turbinado sugar
5 cloves garlic, crushed and peeled or put through a press
5 scallions, thinly sliced
1-inch piece fresh ginger, grated
2 tablespoons canola oil

2 containers firm tofu, drained

Combine marinade ingredients in medium bowl. Add tofu and marinate at least 1 hour. Preheat grill or broiler. Cook tofu for 5 minutes on each side; set aside.

1 package rice sticks
1 package fresh spinach, washed and stems removed
1 lb. green beans or sugar snap peas,
washed and stems removed
¼ cup chopped fresh cilantro

Cook noodles according to directions, until tender. Drain and rinse in warm water; drain well. Transfer to a platter. Arrange the steamed vegetables around the noodles. Slice the tofu and place on top of noodles. Pour marinade over the tofu and top with chopped cilantro.   *Serves 4.*

TEMPEH KABOBS

HIGHLY BENEFICIAL	A, AB	NEUTRAL	O	AVOID	B

These kabobs are great cooked on the barbecue and served over steamed rice or Wild and Basmati Rice Pilaf (see page 193).

1 package tempeh (any variety)

BARBECUE SAUCE

6 oz. plum jam
2 oz. pineapple juice (from the pineapple)
3 tablespoons tamari sauce
2 cloves garlic, put through a press
2 scallions, thinly sliced
2-inch piece fresh ginger, grated

FOR THE SKEWERS

1 large onion, quartered and separated into layers,
2 layers per piece
2 Portobello mushrooms, cut into 1 × 1-inch pieces
2 medium zucchini, cut into 1-inch-thick slices
2 cups 1 × 1-inch pineapple chunks

Prepare grill. Steam tempeh 10 to 15 minutes. Meanwhile, combine barbecue sauce ingredients and prepare vegetables. When the tempeh is cool enough to handle, slice into pieces the same size as the vegetables. Assemble the skewers, alternating vegetables with the tempeh and pineapple. When skewering the zucchini, do so through the green rind. The flesh becomes pulpy when cooked, and won't hold on well. Brush with sauce and grill over medium heat until nicely browned. Serve on a bed of rice. *Serves 4.*

TOFU AND BLACK BEAN CHILI

HIGHLY BENEFICIAL	A	NEUTRAL	O	AVOID	B, AB

A truly fragrant and spicy main course that isn't peppery, but full of freshly ground flavor. The paleness of the tofu contrasts nicely with the black beans.

¼ cup canola or olive oil
2 onions, diced
1 red pepper, diced (TYPE O ONLY)
½ tablespoon ground chili (TYPE O ONLY)
½ tablespoon ground cayenne
1 tablespoon ground coriander
1 tablespoon fresh thyme
1 teaspoon ground cloves
2 tablespoons spelt flour
1 tablespoon sherry
1 container firm tofu, drained and cubed
2 cans black beans, drained and rinsed or 1 cup dried black
beans, soaked overnight and cooked al dente
1 to 1½ cups chicken stock
1 bay leaf
6 cloves garlic, peeled and chopped

In a large pot heat oil over medium heat. Add onions and ground chili and cook 2 minutes, until onions are wilted. Add the remaining spices, stirring well and toasting well to release the flavors. Add the flour and cook 2 more minutes. Be careful not to burn the spice paste. Deglaze with cooking sherry, then add the black beans, stirring well to coat with the spices. Add 1 cup of chicken stock, then the bay leaf and garlic, stirring until incorporated. Simmer 30 minutes, adding more chicken stock as needed. For the last 10 minutes of cooking, add the tofu. Since tofu can be rather fragile, handle it gently, using a wooden spoon. Be sure to remove the bay leaf before serving. Serve with rice or homemade tortillas.   *Serves 4 to 6.*

SILKEN TOFU SCRAMBLE

HIGHLY BENEFICIAL	A, AB	NEUTRAL	O	AVOID	B

Silken is the smoothest, most custardy type of tofu available, and it makes a wonderful substitute for eggs, ricotta cheese, and even yogurt.

1 tablespoon olive oil
1 teaspoon Garlic-Shallot Mixture (see page 334)
1 small carrot, grated
1 small zucchini, grated
5 oz. silken tofu
salt
1 tablespoon chopped fresh parsley or basil

In a small skillet, heat the oil over low heat. Add the shallot-garlic mix and sauté 2 minutes. Add the grated carrot and cook another 3 to 4 minutes. Add the zucchini and silken tofu. With the side of a spoon, chop the tofu as it warms, and stir until cooked. Season with salt and freshly chopped herbs. *Serves 2.*

GRILLED WILD-RICE TEMPEH

HIGHLY BENEFICIAL	A, AB	NEUTRAL	O	AVOID	B

1 package wild-rice tempeh

SIMPLE MARINADE

3 tablespoons olive oil
2 tablespoons tamari sauce

2 tablespoons Garlic-Shallot Mixture (see page 334)
2 tablespoons chopped fresh cilantro
2 tablespoons lemon juice

Remove tempeh from wrapper and place in shallow bowl. In a
small bowl, mix together the remaining ingredients and pour
over the tempeh, turning once. Refrigerate for several hours.
For a quicker marinade, first steam tempeh for 20 minutes,
then marinate 1 hour.

Prepare grill. Cook tempeh over medium heat, turning and basting
with the marinade about 15 minutes, until nicely browned.
Let sit for a few minutes before slicing. Serve with brown rice
pilaf and a crisp romaine salad.   *Serves 4.*

FRUIT–SILKEN TOFU SCRAMBLE

HIGHLY BENEFICIAL	A, AB	NEUTRAL	O	AVOID	B

This alternative breakfast is so delicious, in fact, that it can also
be served as a nutritious desert. Quick and easy to prepare.

TYPE O

2 tablespoons unsalted butter
1 banana, sliced
¼ cup blueberries
8 oz. silken tofu, drained
salt to taste

TYPE A AND TYPE AB

2 tablespoons canola margarine
1 peach, pitted and sliced
¼ cup blueberries

🍴 CYBER RECIPE 🍴

CORN WITH TOFU

THE AUTHOR: Kay A (Alex1Kay@aol.com)

TYPE A

A very quick, easy and great-tasting dish.

3 tablespoons olive oil
16 oz. firm tofu
3 cups fresh sweet corn kernels
1 teaspoon salt
sliced scallions for garnish

Heat the oil in a pot over low heat. Crumble tofu into the pot. Put sweet corn on top of tofu. Cover and cook 3 to 4 minutes, or until tofu is hot and corn is done. Sprinkle a small amount of salt on top of the corn. Mix and serve hot. Just before serving, add scallions as a garnish.
Makes 4 to 6 servings.

8 oz. silken tofu, drained
salt to taste

In a medium skillet, melt butter or margarine over low heat. Add fruit and gently cook 2 to 3 minutes. Let the bananas or peaches caramelize a bit, then add the berries and sauté 2 to 3 minutes. Push the fruit aside and add the silken tofu, chopping and warming it 2 to 3 minutes. The fruit and silken tofu are kept separate so that the tofu doesn't pick up all of the berries' color. At the final minute of cooking, toss them together and add the salt. Serve in a fruit bowl.   *Serves 2.*

BAKED TOFU "FRIES"

HIGHLY BENEFICIAL	A, AB	NEUTRAL	O	AVOID	B

These fries make a tasty sidedish. Serve with Dipping Sauce (see page 335) or Homemade Ketchup (see page 330).

⅓ cup rye cracker crumbs
2 tablespoons quinoa flour
2 tablespoons spices (ground cumin or cayenne,
or oregano and garlic)
1 teaspoon salt
1 cake firm tofu, drained, pressed, and cut into finger-size
sticks

Preheat oven to 350 degrees F. Combine first four ingredients and roll the tofu sticks in the crumb mixture to cover evenly. Brush a cookie sheet with a light coating of oil. Arrange the sticks in a single layer and bake for 35 minutes. Check for crispness, turn over, and bake 10 minutes longer, if necessary. *Serves 2.*

SPICY CURRIED TOFU WITH APRICOTS AND ALMONDS

HIGHLY BENEFICIAL	A	NEUTRAL	O	AVOID	B, AB

Spicy squares of firm tofu are set off by the crunchy almonds and the sweet slivers of dried apricots, which make for a savory and texturally nuanced meal. Serve with a nutty brown rice and a generous portion of steamed broccoli.

SPICY CURRY MARINADE

2 tablespoons tamari sauce
1 tablespoon fresh lemon or lime juice
1 tablespoon chopped fresh parsley or cilantro
1 tablespoon chopped fresh chives
1 tablespoon turbinado sugar
2 teaspoons curry powder
1 teaspoon chili powder (TYPE O ONLY)
1 teaspoon black sesame seeds

1 cake firm tofu, drained and cut into squares

Combine marinade ingredients in a medium bowl. Add tofu cubes, tossing lightly once to coat. Let marinate 1 hour or longer. Meanwhile, prepare the remaining ingredients for the stir-fry.

3 tablespoons olive oil
1 small onion or 3 scallions, sliced
3 carrots, sliced on an angle
2 cloves garlic, peeled and chopped
2 tablespoons water
½ cup sliced dried apricots
⅓ cup sliced almonds

Heat oil in a wok or large skillet over medium-high heat. Add the onion or scallions and sauté 3 minutes. Add the carrots and the garlic and cook 2 minutes, making sure that the garlic doesn't burn. Drain the tofu, and the marinade; set aside. Add tofu to pan and cook until heated through. Add the apricots and almonds, and cook 3 more minutes. Serve over white basmati rice. *Serves 4 to 6.*

NINE

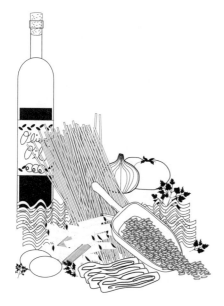

Pasta

INCE MOST PASTA IS MADE OF DURUM SEMOLINA WHEAT flour, many people aren't aware of the wonderful nonwheat varieties. Try rice, buckwheat, Jerusalem artichoke, spelt, quinoa, and spinach pastas. The tastes and textures of these pastas differ considerably from those of the ubiquitous pasta, but they are quite delicious. Sauces also do wonderful things for any pasta. A good sauce can be made from just about anything—the simpler the better.

Spelt flour produces a taste and texture closest to those of traditional pasta. There are two kinds of spelt spaghetti, just as there are two kinds of spelt flour. Like wheat flour, spelt is available in whole grain or white. For the most part, it's always nutritionally beneficial to choose the whole grain. However, the white spelt pasta most resembles the pasta we're all familiar with. If you want a more robust pasta, then the whole-spelt noodles or *soba* buckwheat noodles certainly provide that.

The recipe for pizza pie dough works with both whole-grain or white spelt flour. Be aware that the whole-grain spelt flour doesn't rise as much as the white spelt flour, which doesn't rise as much as white wheat flour.

Some of these recipes mention adding a dusting of pecorino romano or Parmesan, which is the way many people like to eat their pasta. This is optional, although a dusting won't do any harm.

STUFFED SHELLS WITH PESTO

HIGHLY BENEFICIAL	B, AB	NEUTRAL	A	AVOID	O

This pasta, made without tomatoes, is Highly Beneficial to Type B and Type AB, particularly if it's made with rice flour. Semolina or spinach shells are all right; it's the dairy that counts here. Children love these shells, so make plenty of them.

1 lb. shell pasta, either spelt, semolina, or rice flour
1 lb. ricotta cheese
½ lb. mozzarella cheese, grated
½ cup vegetable stock
Basil Pesto (see page 324)

Boil the pasta until done, undercooking by a minute or two, because this dish will cook further once it's assembled. Drain the cooked pasta; set aside. Preheat oven to 375 degrees F.

In a bowl, combine the ricotta and grated mozzarella. Spoon about 1 tablespoon of this mixture into each shell, then place the shells in an oiled glass baking dish, lining them up in neat little rows. When all the shells are filled, pour in the vegetable stock, cover the baking dish with aluminum foil, and bake

about 20 minutes. Remove from oven and serve hot, accompanied by a bowl of pesto to spoon over the shells.
Serves 4 to 6.

GREEN VEGETABLE PASTA

HIGHLY BENEFICIAL		NEUTRAL	O, A	AVOID	B, AB

This beautiful dish is as its name describes—all green. It's a delicious way to incorporate a variety of beneficial vegetables.

> *¼ cup extra-virgin olive oil plus extra for tossing pasta*
> *2 scallions, sliced*
> *1 lb. asparagus, trimmed and cut on the diagonal*
> *into 1-inch pieces*
> *2 green zucchini, sliced on diagonal*
> *4 artichoke hearts, quartered*
> *1 lb. Jerusalem artichoke pasta*
> *salt*
> *¼ cup chopped fresh basil*
> *grated romano cheese*

Bring a large pot of water to a boil. In a large skillet, heat oil over medium heat. Add scallions and cook gently until wilted, about 3 minutes. Add asparagus, zucchini, and artichoke hearts. Cook 3 more minutes. Meanwhile, cook and drain pasta. Rinse well with warm water and drain again. Toss pasta with a little olive oil and season with salt. Cover and keep warm. The vegetables should be tender but still a little crisp. Toss with pasta, sprinkle on the basil, and serve with grated cheese.   *Serves 4.*

SOBA NOODLES OR SPELT PASTA WITH PUMPKIN AND TOFU

HIGHLY BENEFICIAL	A	NEUTRAL	O, AB	AVOID	B

Soba noodles, pumpkin, and tofu are all Highly Beneficial for Type A. Type O and Type AB can substitute rice or spelt pasta. This is a simple dish. Steamed broccoli or a mesclun salad makes a satisfying complement.

olive oil
6 cloves garlic, crushed and peeled
1 medium leek, thinly sliced
water
1 small fresh sugar pumpkin
1 lb. soba noodles or 1 lb. rice or spelt pasta
1 lb. tofu

Put a pot of water on to boil. In a large, heavy skillet, heat 2 tablespoons oil over medium heat. Add garlic and leek, stirring for a few moments. Add ½ cup water, cover, and steam over low heat until leeks are tender, 10 to 15 minutes, adding more water if necessary.

Meanwhile, cut pumpkin in half, remove seeds (save for toasting later), and carefully peel. Cut into 1-inch pieces and add to the skillet with the garlic and leeks. Add an additional ½ cup water and steam pumpkin until tender, 10 to 15 minutes.

The water for the noodles or pasta should be boiling. Add the noodles or pasta and cook according to package directions. When all the vegetables are done, cut the tofu into ½-inch pieces. Add tofu to the skillet and heat thoroughly. Spoon the mixture over the hot noodles. *Serves 4 to 6.*

FETTUCCINE WITH GRILLED LAMB SAUSAGES AND VEGETABLES

HIGHLY BENEFICIAL	B	NEUTRAL	O, AB	AVOID	A

Once the fettuccine is cooked, serve with a simple salad of mixed greens.

> *2 red peppers* (TYPE AB OMIT)
> *2 yellow peppers* (TYPE AB OMIT)
> *2 Portobello mushrooms*
> *2 cloves garlic, crushed and peeled*
> *¼ cup olive oil*
> *1 to 1½ lbs. lamb sausages*
> *1 lb. rice fettuccine*
> *salt*
> *¼ cup chopped fresh basil and parsley*
> *romano cheese*

Prepare grill. Prepare vegetables: Slice peppers in half lengthwise and remove seeds and stems. Remove stems from mushrooms so they lay flat on the grill. Slice eggplants ½-inch thick. Slice zucchini ½-inch thick on diagonal. Rub all of the vegetables with garlic, reserving a small amount, then brush with oil. Grill the lamb sausages over medium-hot coals until nicely browned and juices run clear, about 20 to 25 minutes. Move the sausages to the side of the grill to keep them warm while the vegetables are cooking.

In the meantime, cook the fettuccine in plenty of boiling water. Drain cooked pasta, rinse with warm water, and drain again. Pour remaining olive oil over pasta, and season with salt and pepper. When all the vegetables are nicely grilled, soft but not burned, slice into long strips and toss with garlic. Serve over the fettuccine with a couple of sausages. Sprinkle with fresh herbs and grated romano cheese. *Serves 4.*

GREEN LEAFY PASTA

HIGHLY BENEFICIAL	A	NEUTRAL	O, B, AB	AVOID	

Nutritious leafy greens braised in olive oil and a bit of their own water make a nutritious sauce. Except for the Jerusalem artichoke pasta, this is another all-green meal!

1 lb. spinach pasta (TYPE B AND TYPE AB) *or 1 lb. Jerusalem artichoke pasta* (TYPE O AND TYPE A)
¼ cup olive oil
2 leeks, washed and sliced
2 cloves garlic, chopped
1 bunch spinach, washed and rinsed
1 bunch Swiss chard, washed and trimmed
salt
romano cheese

Bring a large pot of water to a boil. Cook the vegetables as you cook the pasta, drain, and dress with a little oil. Keep covered; the vegetables will be ready soon. In a large skillet, heat oil over medium heat. Add leeks, turning to coat with the oil, and cook them gently several minutes, until they begin to soften and wilt. Add the garlic and stir. A few moments later, add the spinach and Swiss chard, tossing to coat with oil and garlic. The greens will begin to wilt. Steam uncovered several more minutes, or until the greens are fully cooked. Season to taste and grate on some romano. *Serves 4.*

CELLOPHANE NOODLES WITH GRILLED SIRLOIN AND GREEN VEGETABLES

HIGHLY BENEFICIAL	O	NEUTRAL	B	AVOID	A, AB

This is a great dish for company. The Asian-inspired flavors of this dish are refreshing. The bean noodles are light and slippery, absorbing the pungent flavors of the fresh ginger, scallion, and cilantro. Best served at room temperature.

MARINADE

½ cup tamari sauce
⅓ cup rice wine
5 cloves garlic, minced or put through a press
1 tablespoon turbinado sugar
2 scallions, thinly sliced
2 tablespoons olive or canola oil

2 lbs. lean sirloin steak

Combine marinade ingredients. Put steak on large platter. Pour marinade over steak, turning at least once. Marinate for 1 hour, but the longer the better.

cellophane noodles (made from beans)
2 cloves garlic, crushed and peeled
1 lb. sugar snap peas or haricot verte, or delicate string beans, stems removed
1 bunch fresh spinach
Dipping Sauce (see page 335)
¼ cup chopped fresh cilantro
1-inch piece fresh ginger, peeled and grated

While steak is marinating, prepare grill. Drain steak and grill
until medium-rare, about 8 minutes each side; set aside.

Bring a pot of water to a boil for the noodles, and a smaller pot of
water to steam the vegetables. Soften the noodles in hot
water, and then cook according to directions, or until tender.
Rinse in warm water and drain thoroughly. Pile high on platter. Steam garlic and peas for 1 minute or so, then add spinach
and stream 2 more minutes. Arrange the vegetables around
the noodles. Slice the steak, place on top of the noodles, and
drizzle with dipping sauce. Top with fresh cilantro and grated
ginger. *Serves 4.*

PENNE WITH SAUSAGE AND PEPPERS

HIGHLY BENEFICIAL		NEUTRAL	O, B	AVOID	A, AB

This is an updated version of a classic southern Italian dish. Type
B needs to eliminate the tomato sauce. But the dish is just as satisfying "dry." The pasta, of course, is spelt or rice noodles.

8 turkey sausages
¼ cup olive oil
1 large onion thinly sliced
1 tablespoon Garlic-Shallot Mixture (page 334)
or 4 cloves garlic, minced
2 peppers, thinly sliced
¼ cup chopped parsley
2 tablespoons cooking sherry
2 cups tomato sauce (TYPE B OMIT)
salt
1 lb. penne (rice or spelt)

In a heavy skillet brown sausages. When nicely browned, transfer
them to a plate. In the same skillet heat oil over medium heat.

Add onion and Garlic-Shallot Mixture and cook until wilted. Add peppers and parsley and cook a few more minutes, then add sherry. Add tomato sauce and salt to taste. Return sausages to pan and simmer 20 minutes. While sausages are simmering, cook pasta; drain well. Transfer pasta to larger platter. Spoon sausages and peppers over the pasta.   *Serves 4.*

SAUTÉED VEGETABLES WITH QUINOA PASTA

HIGHLY BENEFICIAL	A, AB	NEUTRAL	O	AVOID	B

Although this pasta appears to be neutral for all blood types it's not always. It cannot be stressed enough how important it is to *read the labels on all packaged items.* Quinoa pasta found in the stores usually lists corn flour as the first ingredient, then quinoa flour. It's wonderfully tasty and quite yellow—a dead giveaway to its origins—but it's suitable only for Type A. All other blood types should use a beneficial pasta, such as spelt, buckwheat, or rice.

¼ cup olive oil
4 cloves garlic, crushed and peeled
¼ cup chopped fresh parsley
2 Portobello mushrooms, thinly sliced
¼ cup sherry
1 container firm tofu (optional)
1 small head radicchio, washed and sliced
1 bunch dandelion greens, broccoli rabe, or spinach,
washed well and tough stems removed
salt
1 lb. rice pasta
olive oil (for pasta)
romano cheese (optional, according to blood type)

Boil water for the pasta. In a very large skillet, heat the oil over low heat and gently cook the garlic, being sure not to darken the cloves, which will make them bitter. Add parsley and cook 2 minutes. Add mushrooms and cook until soft, about 5 minutes. Add sherry, and cook 1 minute to burn off the alcohol. Add tofu, if using, radicchio, and greens. The volume will seem unmanageable at first, but it will quickly reduce. Turn the greens over as they cook, so that the somewhat wilted bottoms are on top. Cover and cook 10 minutes. Season with salt to taste. Meanwhile, add the pasta to the water and cook according to directions. Drain and rinse with warm water. Toss with a little olive oil to keep it from sticking. Place the pasta on the plate first, then smother with the vegetables. Top with grated romano cheese. *Serves 4.*

COLD SOBA NOODLES WITH THAI PEANUT SAUCE

HIGHLY BENEFICIAL	A	NEUTRAL		AVOID	O, B, AB

1 package buckwheat (soba) noodles
1 cup Peanut Butter Sauce (see page 330)
2 cups shredded romaine, washed and dried
1 cup grated carrots
2 scallions, thinly sliced
chopped fresh cilantro

Cook noodles in plenty of water according to package directions. Drain, then rinse in tepid water and drain again. Toss with sauce. On a platter or 2 serving plates, spread the lettuce, then the shredded carrots. Roll noodles on top. Sprinkle with sliced scallion and fresh cilantro and serve. *Serves 2.*

BROCCOLI RABE WITH PASTA

HIGHLY BENEFICIAL		NEUTRAL	O, A, B, AB	AVOID	

The slightly bitter broccoli rabe, the sharp romano cheese, and the pungent garlic interact to produce strong, clear flavors. Rice flour makes a sturdy pasta, with a texture similar to that of regular spaghetti. Whole spelt, on the other hand, resembles buckwheat noodles. The whole-spelt pasta has a coarser grain, so an earthier texture. The shorter rice pastas are more delicate than the longer versions. Whichever you choose, be sure to cook it in plenty of water, stir frequently, and lightly rinse it with warm water after cooking.

The degree of doneness can sometimes be a problem. If you cook any pasta for too long, it can become a soggy mush. Rice noodles and spelt pasta are not exceptions. *Al dente*, or slightly firm, is the preferred texture. Keep sampling individual strands as the pasta nears completion. When the texture feels right to you, it's done. Drain and rinse, then top with the cooked rabe and serve.

3 tablespoons olive oil
2 tablespoons Garlic-Shallot Mixture (see page 334)
1 bunch rappini, washed and trimmed
2 to 3 tablespoons water
1 package spelt pasta
2 tablespoons tamari
salt
freshly shaved pecorino romano cheese

Boil a pot of water to cook the pasta. Heat 2 tablespoons oil in a large skillet over medium heat. Add garlic mixture and cook 1 minute. Cut the very tip of the stems from broccoli rabe and discard. Cut remaining rabe in thirds. Place in skillet and cook for a few minutes, turning once. Add 2 tablespoons water, cover, and cook another few minutes. Put pasta into boiling water and stir well; return to a boil and stir again. The pasta will take about 5 to 7 minutes. At this point, check the broccoli rabe. If tender, remove from skillet and and set aside. Drain pasta and toss with remaining tablespoon oil and salt to taste. Serve pasta topped with rabe and grated romano cheese. *Serves 4.*

SPAGHETTI AND MEAT SAUCE

HIGHLY BENEFICIAL		NEUTRAL	O	AVOID	A, B, AB

For a quick, delicious meal, spaghetti and meat sauce is right on the mark. This recipe takes almost no time to make if you have homemade sauce, or if you have a jar of organic tomato sauce on hand. The jar sauces have become increasingly more sophisticated, and they certainly take a lot less time than preparing sauce from scratch.

1 lb. ground organic beef
4 tablespoons olive oil
1 medium onion, diced
1 red pepper, diced
2 cups tomato sauce
sprig of rosemary
1 package rice spaghetti
pinch of salt
romano cheese

Boil a pot of water to cook the pasta. In a large skillet, brown beef; drain well and reserve. In same skillet, heat 3 tablespoons oil over medium heat and cook onion and pepper until it is soft. Return meat to skillet, add tomato sauce and rosemary, and cook on low heat until pasta is done. Cook spaghetti, stirring frequently, before and after it reaches a boil. Drain well and lightly rinse with warm water. Toss with remaining 1 tablespoon olive oil and a pinch of salt. Serve sauce over pasta, with a dusting of grated romano.   *Serves 4.*

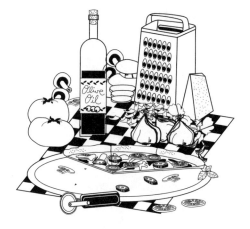

Pizza

IZZA IS A WAY OF LIFE IN SOME HOUSEHOLDS.
There's nothing you can't put on a homemade pizza. Admittedly,
it's a lot more work to make your own pizza than it is to call for a
takeout version, but please don't hold the Blood Type Diet responsible for that. We wish that local pizzerias made spelt pizzas!
The pizza dough recipe we're offering you is really very easy.
The basic dough can be topped with a multitude of toppings as
well as tomato sauce and mozzarella cheese. For Type A and
Type B, the concept of a traditional pizza without the tomato
sauce has to be modified. Who says you can't make what's known
as a "white" pizza? Who says you can't use soy cheese and other
Highly Beneficial Type A and Type B foods instead? Just a few
years ago someone came up with the idea for a salad pizza, which
really does have its place in the diets of an awful lot of people!

BASIC PIZZA DOUGH

HIGHLY BENEFICIAL		NEUTRAL	O, A, B, AB	AVOID	

This is a light, thin, whole-grain pizza dough. For a more traditional pizza dough, you can substitute all-white spelt for the whole-grain spelt flour. This yields two 12-inch pies.

1 tablespoon dry yeast
1 cup warm water (warm to the wrist)
2½ to 3 cups flour (1½ cups white spelt,
plus 1½ cups whole spelt)
2 tablespoons olive oil
scant teaspoon salt
olive oil for the bowl

In a large mixing bowl, dissolve the yeast in warm water. Add 1½ cups flour and mix well with a large spoon. Add oil, salt, and the rest of the flour and work into a manageable dough. Turn onto a well-floured surface and knead for 5 minutes, adding more flour as the dough gets sticky. Wash out the same bowl and grease with olive oil. Put the dough back into the bowl and turn once to cover with oil. Cover with a clean kitchen towel, and let rise for 1 hour. Once the dough has doubled in size, punch it down and divide it into 2 pieces. On a flat work area, roll the dough briefly for 1 minute and set aside to relax in a bowl or on a sheet pan for 15 minutes.

Preheat oven to 475 degrees F and sprinkle a rectangular baking sheet or a classic round pizza pan with a wisp of cornmeal to keep the pizza from sticking. It's worth investing the money for a pizza pan. They don't cost much and are handy in other ways in the kitchen. Take 1 ball of dough and flatten and press with your fingers, coaxing it to fit the pan. Brush with olive oil. Add toppings. See following recipes.

CALIFORNIA PIZZA

HIGHLY BENEFICIAL		NEUTRAL	O, AB	AVOID	A, B

1 basic dough (see page 178), ½ recipe
3 tablespoons tomato sauce
½ lb. mozzarella, sliced
2 teaspoons grated romano
2 tablespoons goat cheese, crumbled
2 tablespoons chopped fresh basil
olive oil

Follow the general directions for pizza dough. Preheat oven to 475 degrees F. Spread dough with tomato sauce. Top with mozzarella, grated romano, and goat cheese. Sprinkle with basil and drizzle with olive oil. Bake in middle of preheated oven at least 10 minutes. Keep an eye on it. Let cool 5 to 8 minutes before serving.   *Serves 2 to 3.*

SALAD PIZZA

HIGHLY BENEFICIAL		NEUTRAL	O, A, B, AB	AVOID	

1 basic dough (see page 178), ½ recipe
olive oil
about 2 cups mesclun salad
½ small red onion, chopped
Olive Oil & Lemon Dressing (see page 326)
grated romano, crumbled feta, Roquefort, or Gruyère
½ teaspoon dried oregano

Follow the general directions for pizza dough. Preheat oven to 475 degrees F. Brush dough with olive oil. Bake until golden

🍴 C Y B E R   R E C I P E 🍴

PIZZA SAUCE SUBSTITUTE
AUTHOR: Susan (byrandsu@pacbell.net)

TYPE B

Yummy sauce for homemade pizza and you won't miss the tomato! This sauce works like a charm, and my pizza-loving Type O raves over it.

2 teaspoons sugar
1 teaspoon salt
2 teaspoons paprika
1 teaspoon powdered oregano
1 teaspoon dried basil
1 teaspoon dried thyme
2 teaspoons dried parsley
2 teaspoon onion powder
1 teaspoon garlic powder
3 drops anise flavoring
½ cup water

Working in a small bowl, mix dry spices and powders. Stir in anise flavoring. Stir in water. Looks just like spaghetti sauce! With a rubber spatula, spread a THIN layer on the pizza dough, concentrating it slightly around the edge, then add your toppings and bake as usual. The sauce is very highly flavored, so a little goes a long way.
Makes sauce for 1 medium pizza.

brown. It may puff up a bit; just poke it with a fork. Lightly toss the salad with onion and dressing. Allow to wilt. Top the baked crust with the salad and oregano, and sprinkle with grated cheese. *Serves 2 to 4.*

WHITE PIZZA

HIGHLY BENEFICIAL		NEUTRAL	O, A, B, AB	AVOID	

White pizza is as delicious as the traditional tomato-based pizza and is adaptable to all blood types. The toppings for white pizza are many, varied, and delicious. These pizzas aren't the thick, drippy ones from the corner pizza parlor. In fact, in their form and flavor, they closely resemble true Northern Italian *pizze*. The Italians prefer thin crusts, few toppings, and a light hand with cheese. These are always garnished with extra-virgin olive oil. Try some of these interesting combinations and see for yourself how really good these homemade *pizze* can be!

ARTICHOKE HEARTS AND ONIONS

HIGHLY BENEFICIAL		NEUTRAL	O, A	AVOID	B, AB

1 basic dough (see page 178), ½ recipe
3 tablespoons extra-virgin olive oil
1 medium onion, thinly sliced
4 cooked artichoke hearts, thinly sliced
4 oz. low-fat mozzarella, grated
2 oz. goat cheese, crumbled
2 tablespoons chopped Italian parsley

Follow the general directions for pizza dough. Preheat oven to 475 degrees F. In a skillet, heat 2 tablespoons oil over medium heat. Add onion and sauté until it softens, about 5 minutes. Let cool slightly, then spread the onion over the dough. Place sliced artichoke hearts around the top, and cover with mozzarella and crumbled goat cheese. Sprinkle with chopped parsley and drizzle with remaining oil. Bake 10 to 15 minutes, or until crust looks golden brown. Remove from oven and let cool for 5 minutes before serving.   *Serves 2 to 4.*

ZUCCHINI AND BASIL PIZZA

HIGHLY BENEFICIAL		NEUTRAL	O, A, B, AB	AVOID	

1 basic dough (see page 178), ½ recipe
2 medium-size green zucchini
2 medium-size yellow squash
½ teaspoon salt
2 tablespoons Garlic-Shallot Mixture (see page 334)
¼ cup grated pecorino romano cheese
¼ cup fresh basil, chopped
1 tablespoon extra-virgin olive oil

Follow the general directions for pizza dough. Preheat oven to 475 degrees F. Wash and dry all the squash. Slice on a long angle, about ¼ inch thick. Lay the zucchini out on paper towels and sprinkle with salt. Brush the dough with Garlic-Shallot Mixture. Blot moisture from basil and zucchini. Layer zucchini slices evenly around the top of the dough, alternating green with yellow, until the surface has been covered. Top with grated cheese and basil, and drizzle with oil. Bake 15 to 20 minutes on the top rack of the oven until crust is browned and squash is cooked.   *Serves 2 to 4.*

SPINACH AND RICOTTA PIZZA

HIGHLY BENEFICIAL		NEUTRAL	A, B, AB	AVOID	O

1 basic dough (see page 178), ½ recipe
1 bunch fresh spinach, washed, dried, and chopped

1 cup low-fat ricotta cheese
2 tablespoons fresh garlic, put through a press
1 to 1½ teaspoons salt
2 tablespoons chopped fresh parsley or basil
⅓ cup grated pecorino romano cheese
1 cup grated mozzarella cheese
1 tablespoon olive oil

Follow the general directions for pizza dough. Preheat oven to 475 degrees F. Carefully wash the fresh spinach to remove all grit, and then lightly steam until wilted. Mix spinach with ricotta, garlic, salt, and parsley or basil. Spread mixture evenly over dough. Top with grated cheeses and drizzle with olive oil. Bake on a lower rack 10 to 15 minutes, or until golden brown. *Serves 2 to 4.*

POTATO-ONION PIZZA

HIGHLY BENEFICIAL		NEUTRAL	B, AB	AVOID	O, A

1 basic dough (see page 178), ½ recipe
2 tablespoons olive oil
6 to 8 small red potatoes, steamed and cooled
1 small red onion, sliced thinly
rosemary
4 to 6 oz. Gruyère, grated
salt

Follow the general directions for pizza dough. Preheat oven to 475 degrees F. Lightly steam the spinach, and then combine with the ricotta. Slice the cooked red potatoes into slivers and arrange over the dough. Top with sliced onion. Season with rosemary and salt. Top with grated cheese. Bake 10 to 15 minutes, or until crust is golden brown. *Serves 2 to 4.*

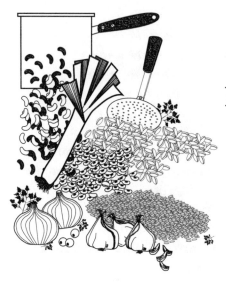

ELEVEN

Beans & Grains

Legumes *aka* Beans

LEGUMES ARE PLANTS that produce edible seeds within a pod. Legumes constitute an enormous family with more than six hundred genuses and thirteen thousand species. Beans, broad beans, soybeans, peas, lentils, and peanuts are all legumes. They provide a sizable amount of protein and some complex carbohydrates. Unlike animal proteins, legumes are incomplete proteins, lacking some of the essential amino acids. However, many cultures rely heavily on legumes as their primary source of protein, instinctively combining them with grains and some dairy products to gain all of the essential amino acids necessary to form complete proteins.

For many people, beans cause considerable difficulty during digestion, leading to flatulence and intestinal discomfort. Some beans cause worse distress than others. If you don't regularly consume beans, start slowly and cautiously. Preparation is the key to success. When soaking beans, drain them every few hours and add fresh water to continue soaking off the enzymes that are the source of the bean's digestive aftereffects. Use fresh water when you cook the beans. Drain and rinse canned beans well. And be sure to cook dried beans thoroughly! They must be tender. Cook them longer than you might otherwise, even if you are following directions. Many things can affect the cooking time of beans, such as the age of the beans, type of water, altitude, and where the beans were grown. Eat a small amount. Start with a tablespoon or two with a grain dish such as rice.

LIMA BEANS WITH GOAT CHEESE AND SCALLIONS

HIGHLY BENEFICIAL	B	NEUTRAL	O	AVOID	A, AB

Lima beans are neutral benefit for Type O and are highly beneficial for Type B. They're very creamy with a mild flavor. They're so creamy, in fact, that they're often referred to as butter beans. Don't overcook lima beans; they turn mushy very quickly once they've softened. Also, be aware that cooking lima beans produces a lot of foam, so they're not necessarily the best bet for a pressure cooker. They can make a delicious main-course salad, with a lemon vinaigrette dressing—Types B and AB can have oil and vinegar—and sprinkled with goat cheese and scallions.

*1 package frozen baby limas or 1 cup dried lima beans or 2
cups fresh lima beans
1 tablespoon olive oil
2 scallions, thinly sliced
2 cloves garlic, crushed and peeled
dressing of choice*

4 oz. goat cheese
3 tablespoons fresh parsley, minced

Prepare lima beans and put them in a serving bowl. In a skillet, heat oil over medium to high heat. Add the scallions and sauté a minute or two until fragrant. Add garlic, turning briefly until it just begins to color. Add scallions and garlic to the lima beans. Pour 2 to 3 tablespoons of dressing over the beans and toss gently. Crumble goat cheese over the top and garnish with parsley. Serve at room temperature.   *Serves 4.*

BLACK-EYED PEAS WITH LEEKS

HIGHLY BENEFICIAL	O, A	NEUTRAL		AVOID	B, AB

If you use canned beans, or if you plan ahead and soak some the night before, this is an easy, delicious dish, served either hot or cold. Serve it hot with rice for dinner or cold (or room-temperature) with a dressing of olive oil and lemon juice for a quick lunch.

2 cups cooked black-eyed peas
1 tablespoon olive oil
1 small leek, thinly sliced
1 clove garlic, crushed and peeled
¼ cup water
pinch of salt
¼ cup fresh cilantro, chopped

Put the beans in a pot to heat. In a cast-iron skillet, heat oil over low heat. Add leek and garlic, turning well to coat with oil. Add water, cover, and braise leek until soft. Add more water as needed, 1 tablespoon at a time. When leek is tender, add it to the beans and heat thoroughly. Toss gently with cilantro and salt.   *Serves 4.*

LENTIL SALAD

HIGHLY BENEFICIAL	A, AB	NEUTRAL		AVOID	O, B

This lentil salad tastes great, and is an excellent accompaniment to other, interesting ingredients. This is a slightly "sweet" salad that is perfect for lunch and dinner.

2 cup lentils
8 cups water
½ cup dried cherries
½ cup raisins
½ cup walnuts, broken into pieces
2 tablespoons olive oil
juice of ½ lemon
pinch of salt

Cook the lentils in the water, gently simmering, until done, 30 to 40 minutes. Start checking at 30 minutes because lentils can overcook very quickly. Drain and let cool. Add cherries, raisins, and walnuts. Whisk together oil, lemon, and salt. Pour dressing over salad, mixing gently and thoroughly. *Serves 4 to 6.*

PURÉED PINTO BEANS WITH GARLIC

HIGHLY BENEFICIAL	O, A, AB	NEUTRAL		AVOID	B

With brown rice and braised kale, these beans make a very filling and quick dinner. Also try this as a different and delicious dip for raw vegetables.

2 tablespoons olive oil
1 medium onion, diced

6 cloves garlic, crushed
1 can pinto beans, drained and rinsed, or 1 cup
dry pinto beans, soaked and cooked
1 teaspoon ground cumin (or to taste)
generous pinch of salt
3 tablespoons chopped fresh cilantro

In a cast-iron skillet, heat 2 tablespoons oil over very low heat. Add diced onion and cook about 10 minutes, stirring frequently, until onion is golden brown. Add garlic and sauté a few minutes more. Add beans and spices, then cook another few minutes. Transfer mixture to blender and purée until very smooth. You might have to scrape down the blender once or twice to get it all. Serve sprinkled with the cilantro.   *Serves 4.*

Grains

THERE IS A very wide variety of life-sustaining grains. Today, long forgotten or ignored grains such as spelt and quinoa have been rediscovered and are being cultivated. For people with wheat intolerance, alternative grains are a real boon, whether these grains are used as flours in breads, pastas, and cereals or as whole grains cooked like buckwheat or rice. Many of these rediscovered grains have unfamiliar tastes and textures, which make them exciting and different. There's a world of grains to discover.

Rice

HIGHLY BENEFICIAL	AB	NEUTRAL	O, A, B	AVOID	

The second largest food crop in the world behind wheat, rice has almost eight thousand varieties. Wild rice belongs to a different species altogether. Rice is an extraordinarily compatible grain that can be enjoyed by all blood types. There are many kinds of rice sold under various trademarks: basmati, Texmati™, wild pecan, Lundberg Royal™, Wehani™, Black Japonica™, Jasmati™, arborio, white and brown sushi, short- and long-grain white and brown, sweet brown, and many others.

Mixed–blood type families as well as guests always appreciate a main course with rice. The rule of thumb is 2 cups of water to 1 cup rice. Allow about 20 to 25 minutes of cooking time for white rice, and 35 to 40 minutes for brown rice.

Wild Rice

HIGHLY BENEFICIAL	AB	NEUTRAL	O, A	AVOID	B

Not a rice at all but an aquatic grass, wild rice is truly a native American crop, the uncultivated varieties of which grow in the wetlands around many northern lakes and rivers. Wild rice has a more complex taste and aroma than those of most grains, and its beautiful, dark color and crunchy texture set it apart from domesticated grains. Wild rice is now grown commercially in California, but there are those who still prefer the hand-harvested wild rice.

Because of its variations, it is hard to gauge the amount of water needed to cook wild rice. For 1 cup wild rice, begin with 2 to 2½ cups water and keep an eye on it. Bring to a boil, then reduce heat to low. The rice is done when it's tender and some of the individual grains have burst open. Add more water, a tablespoon at a time, or cook the rice a little longer to absorb the last of the water.

Amaranth

HIGHLY BENEFICIAL	A	NEUTRAL	O, AB	AVOID	B

A tiny grain from a majestic, maroon-headed plant, amaranth was a staple food of the Aztecs. It is high in protein, calcium, phosphorus, iron, and fiber as well as the amino acids lysine and methionine. Toast these seeds lightly before cooking by tossing the seeds in a preheated cast-iron pan over a medium-low heat. Allow 1 cup of amaranth to 1 cup water.

Buckwheat

HIGHLY BENEFICIAL	A	NEUTRAL	O	AVOID	B, AB

Buckwheat originated in Asia, and it is actually a seed rather than a true grain. Buckwheat is high in protein, B vitamins, vitamin E, iron, and calcium. It is best known as kasha, a hearty porridge, and it also makes an excellent pancake. Buckwheat can also substitute for corn and makes a wonderfully rich and different polenta.

Kamut

HIGHLY BENEFICIAL		NEUTRAL	O, A	AVOID	B, AB

An ancient Egyptian grain, kamut is a distant relative of modern hybrid wheat. It contains far more protein than wheat while being far less allergen-producing. The kernels are larger than wheat berries and have a nutty taste and smooth texture. Kamut resembles rice in shape and is a good choice for salads and pilafs.

Millet

HIGHLY BENEFICIAL	B, AB	NEUTRAL	O, A	AVOID	

One of the most ancient of grains, common millet is grown in China, India, Russia, southern Europe, and parts of North America. Foxtail millet is among China's five most sacred crops. There is no one millet—the name is given to a number of cereal grains that don't even belong in the same genus. Pearl millet is cultivated in India; sorghum in India, Africa, and China. Another strain of millet is cultivated in the Philippines as well as in Ethiopia, where it's called *teff* and is the essential ingredient of *injera,* the Ethiopian flatbread. In its various forms it has been eaten as a porridge for millennia. Millet has been grown as a grain to stave off famine, because it is so hardy and grows in such inhospitable environments. Rich in phosphorus, iron, calcium, riboflavin, and niacin, it also contains the amino acid lysine, something which cornmeal doesn't. Eaten in combination with tofu or beans, millet forms a complete protein.

Quinoa

HIGHLY BENEFICIAL		NEUTRAL	O, A, B, AB	AVOID	

The tiny quinoa seed contains a germ with far more protein than any other grain, and of higher quality. Its amino acids are more balanced than those of other grains, with high levels of lysine, methionine, and cystine. Not really a grain at all, quinoa's genus can be found in the herb family. It was a sacred food of the Incas for centuries. It ideally complements beans for a complete protein meal. Among its many recommendations, quinoa is a source of iron, magnesium, zinc, copper, potassium, riboflavin, thiamin, niacin, and phosphorus. Quinoa has reemerged from obscurity and is finding its way into more people's diets every day. Quinoa's high protein and low gluten contents, nutty flavor, and crunchy texture make it a worthwhile addition to anyone's diet, particularly since it can readily substitute for most other grains, and its reaction is neutral for all blood types.

Spelt

HIGHLY BENEFICIAL		NEUTRAL	O, A, B, AB	AVOID	

A nonhybridized wheat that was a staple in biblical times, spelt will soon become a modern-day staple, not only for its nonallergenic properties, but for its great nutritive value. Spelt contains more protein, amino acids, B vitamins, and minerals than does its distant cousin, hybridized wheat. Spelt is available in many different forms. Whole-spelt and white-spelt flours can be substituted pretty closely for any wheat recipe, and pastas made from spelt are good replacements for durum and semolina, although the current cost is three times higher than that of wheat products. Whole-spelt flour makes for a denser dough than white-spelt flour, which is still slightly denser than that made from commercial white flour. Spelt berries are large, moist, slightly chewy, and flavorful, similar in texture to barley. The spelt berries make excellent grain salads.

FARO PILAF

HIGHLY BENEFICIAL		NEUTRAL	O, A, B, AB	AVOID	

Faro is the Italian word for "spelt," and it makes a different, nuttier alternative to rice in this recipe for pilaf.

1 cup faro
2 cups water
olive oil
3 cloves garlic, crushed and peeled
2 small zucchini, diced small
2 tablespoons fresh parsley, chopped
salt
pecorino romano cheese

Combine faro and water in a saucepan and bring to a boil. Reduce heat, cover, and steam until all water is absorbed, about 20 minutes. Meanwhile, heat about 2 tablespoons oil in a heavy cast-iron skillet over medim-low heat. Add garlic and sauté a few moments. Add zucchini and stir until coated with oil. Cover and steam until soft, about 5 to 8 minutes. Add parsley, cover pan, and allow to steam another minute. Remove from heat and place in bowl with faro; mix together. Add salt to taste. Grate a little pecorino romano over the dish. *Serves 3 to 4.*

WILD AND BASMATI RICE PILAF

HIGHLY BENEFICIAL	AB	NEUTRAL	O, A	AVOID	B

The following recipe is easy to prepare, as it calls for the most basic of ingredients and a modest cooking time.

1 cup wild rice, cooked in 2 to 3 cups water
1 cup basmati rice, cooked in 2 cups water
3 green scallions, sliced
¼ cup olive oil
2 teaspoons salt

Cook the rices in separate pans. When the rices are cooked, combine them, toss with the scallions and olive oil, and salt to taste. *Serves 4 to 6.*

MILLET TABBOULEH

| HIGHLY BENEFICIAL | B, AB | NEUTRAL | O, A | AVOID | |

Millet's versatility makes it a perfect choice for recipes calling for bulghur wheat. Traditionally, tabbouleh is a parsley and mint salad with the occasional sprinkling of grain. Here we have replaced the traditional cracked bulghur with millet. Feel free to increase the fresh herbs as desired.

> *2½ cups water (vegetable stock makes for more flavor)*
> *1 cup millet, lighly toasted without oil*
> *3 scallions, thinly sliced*
> *1 cucumber, peeled, seeded, and diced small*
> *3 plum tomatoes, chopped (optional)*
> *¼ cup chopped fresh parsley*
> *¼ cup chopped fresh mint*
> *2 tablespoons olive oil*
> *1 juice of lemon*
> *salt*

Bring water to a boil. Add millet, stir, and return to boil. Reduce heat and summer 15 to 20 minutes, or until all water is absorbed. Let sit off heat 10 minutes. Transfer cooked millet to a bowl and let cool slightly. Add scallions, cucumber, tomatoes, if using, parsley, and mint; mix well. Dress with oil and lemon. Add salt to taste. *Serves 3 to 4.*

MILLET COUSCOUS

HIGHLY BENEFICIAL	B, AB	NEUTRAL	O, A	AVOID	

Couscous is not just a grain, but the name of the national dish of North African countries such as Algeria, Morocco, and Tunisia. It is produced from semolina, the flour that results from the milling of the endosperm of hard durum wheat. Couscous is produced by mixing the resulting semolina with flour and sprinkling the two with cold salted water. It is then rolled and pressed (usually by hand) to produce the tiny beads of couscous. This variation of the traditional couscous is made from the ubiquitous millet, and is quite good eaten on its own, though it marries easily with vegetables, meats, soups, stews, or salads. This recipe uses the millet couscous as part of a deliciously textured salad.

1 cup millet, lightly toasted without oil
2½ cups water or vegetable stock
2 carrots, diced small
1 small red onion, diced small
¼ cup raisins, plumped (by soaking in hot water)
3 tablespoons sunflower seeds (TYPES O, A) *or 3 tablespoons*
chopped walnuts (TYPES O, B, AND AB)
2 tablespoons olive oil
1 juice of lemon
salt

Cook millet and transfer to a bowl. Add carrots, red onions, raisins, and sunflower seeds or walnuts. Whisk together the olive oil and lemon juice and pour over the millet. Add salt to taste. Also quite good when topped with silken tofu. *Serves 3 to 4.*

SPELT BERRY AND BASMATI RICE PILAF

HIGHLY BENEFICIAL		NEUTRAL	O, A, B, AB	AVOID	

The chewy spelt berries give this pilaf additional body and flavor.

1 cup cooked spelt berries
1 cup cooked basmati rice (increase amount of rice if desired)
2 scallions, diced
2 tablespoons olive oil
salt

Combine all ingredients and let sit for at least 15 minutes. Serve at room temperature.   *Serves 4.*

SPELT BERRY AND RICE SALAD

HIGHLY BENEFICIAL	AB	NEUTRAL	O, B	AVOID	A

This is a slighly different version of the pilaf recipe offered previously. The colors alone make for an appealing dish, but the taste and textures add their own interesting note.

1 cup cooked spelt berries
1 to 2 cups cooked rice (any variety)
1 yellow pepper, diced small (TYPE AB SUBSTITUTE 1 CUP
SAUTÉED MAITAKE MUSHROOMS)
3 tablespoons chopped fresh parsley
1 tablespoon diced jalapeño peppers (TYPE AB OMIT)
3 tablespoons olive oil
salt

Combine all ingredients and serve at room temperature. Feel
free to add scallions, garlic, and complementary spices such as
coriander and a dusting of cumin. The dish can hold in the refrigerator up to 4 days.   *Serves 4 to 5.*

QUINOA RISOTTO

HIGHLY BENEFICIAL		NEUTRAL	O, A, B, AB	AVOID	

Traditional Italian risotto is cooked with the classic round rice
known as *arborio.* The rice is first cooked in oil or butter for a few
minutes while being constantly stirred. Liquid is added, and then
the mixture is simmered until the liquid is absorbed. Cooked in
this manner, the rice remains separate and firm. Using quinoa in
place of the rice doesn't change the essential texture of the dish
and adds a tremendous protein boost to the meal, as quinoa contains far more protein than do most other grains.

> *2 tablespoons olive oil*
> *1 onion, diced*
> *2 cloves garlic, minced*
> *1 red pepper, minced* (Types O and B only)
> *3 tablespoons chopped fresh flat-leaf parlsey*
> *2 cups quinoa, rinsed and drained*
> *3¼ cups vegetable broth*
> *salt*

Heat oil in a medium saucepan over medim heat. Add the onion
and garlic and cook a few minutes, being careful not to burn
the garlic. Add the red pepper and parsley and continue cooking another minute. Add the quinoa and cook a few moments,
thoroughly coating the quinoa with the oil and vegetables,
then add the stock. Water may be used, although vegetable
broth adds flavor to the dish. Bring to a boil, then reduce to a

simmer, cover, and cook 15 minutes. Season with salt to taste. Serve immediately. This dish is good served cold.   *Serves 4.*

BROWN RICE PILAF

HIGHLY BENEFICIAL	AB	NEUTRAL	O, A, B	AVOID	

Any brown rice will do for this pilaf, but brown basmati rice has a slightly nutty flaor that is quite pleasing. Some of the colored rices added in any proportion to the brown rice also provide variations in texture and are quite decorative.

1 cup brown rice
2 cups water
2 tablespoons olive oil
4 cloves garlic, crushed and peeled
1 large carrot, diced
½ cup water
¼ cup fresh cilantro, chopped
salt

Combine rice and 2 cups water in a saucepan and bring to a boil. Reduce heat, cover, and steam 40 minutes, or until all water has been absorbed. Always check your rice toward the end of the cooking time. Rice cooking times are specific to the variety and will vary. While the rice cooks, heat 2 tablespoons oil in a heavy skillet over medium heat. Add garlic and sauté gently a few moments. Add carrot, stir to coat with oil, and add remaining ½ cup water. Reduce heat, cover pan, and simmer until carrot is tender but not soft. Check carefully to be sure there is sufficient water to braise the carrot, adding water in small quantities if necessary. Add coriander in the last few minutes, letting it steam. When rice is cooked, place carrot and rice in bowl, mixing gently. Add salt to taste.   *Serves 4.*

WILD RICE SALAD

HIGHLY BENEFICIAL	AB	NEUTRAL	O, A	AVOID	B

Here's a chance to use wild rice in a festive and interesting way. This is a very pretty dish that makes an admirable accompaniment to squab, Cornish game hens, lamb, and venison.

1 cup hand-harvested wild rice
1 cup dried apricots, diced
1 cup walnuts, chopped
1 cup dried cherries
¼ cup olive oil
juice of 1 lemon
1 tablespoon maple syrup
salt

Bring 3 cups water to a boil. Add wild rice. Cover, reduce heat, and simmer about 45 minutes, or until tender. Drain any remaining water and reserve for stock. Toss rice lightly with fork. Plump dried apricots by pouring boiling water over them; let sit until soft. When rice has cooled for a while, add walnuts, cherries, and apricots, mixing well. Whisk together olive oil, lemon juice, maple syrup, and pinch of salt. Pour over salad, turning well. Adjust seasoning to taste. The wild rice salad tastes best when served at room temperature.
Serves 3 to 4.

SPELT BERRY SALAD

HIGHLY BENEFICIAL		NEUTRAL	O, A, B, AB	AVOID	

Spelt berries suit all of the blood types. Make this salad for lunch, or serve it with fish or tofu for dinner.

1 cup spelt berries
1 cucumber, peeled and diced
2 scallions, finely sliced
¼ cup red onion, finely chopped
¼ cup fresh cilantro, chopped
2 tablespoons olive oil
juice of 1 lemon
salt
2 tablespoons crumbled goat cheese

Cook spelt in 4 cups water about 45 minutes, until tender and chewy. Add cucumber, scallions, red onion, and cilantro and mix gently. Dress with olive oil, lemon juice, and salt to taste. Sprinkle with goat cheese. *Serves 4.*

Combinations: Beans and Grains

THERE ARE ENDLESS combinations of beans and grains, which means there is a wide variety of wonderful cold dishes. The possibilities are virtually limitless! Add a combination of fresh or cooked vegetables, some fresh herbs, olive oil, cheese, and spices. Don't be afraid to try different things.

BLACK-EYED PEAS AND BARLEY SALAD

HIGHLY BENEFICIAL	O, A	NEUTRAL		AVOID	B, AB

This recipe is simple, and so easy to make. Combine with some fresh steamed vegetables. Serve any leftovers the very next day for a quick lunch.

1 cup cooked black-eyed peas (if canned, rinse and drain)
1 cup cooked barley
½ red onion, diced small
2 tablespoons chopped fresh cilantro
1 tablespoon salt
2 tablespoons olive oil
1 tablespoon diced jalapeño pepper (TYPE O)
½ cup cooked corn (TYPE A)

Combine all ingredients, toss gently and thoroughly, and let flavors meld for a while before serving. *Serves 4.*

SOY BEANS, KAMUT, AND BASMATI RICE

HIGHLY BENEFICIAL		NEUTRAL	O, A	AVOID	B, AB

Kamut and basmati rice make a wonderfully nutty-tasting combination, while the addition of the soy beans makes this a complete protein dish.

1 cup cooked kamut
1 cup cooked soy beans
1 cup cooked basmati rice
½ cooked yellow squash
3 tablespoons extra-virgin olive oil

3 tablespoons chopped fresh cilantro
½ teaspoon chopped jalapeño pepper (TYPE O ONLY)
salt

Combine all the cooked grains and legumes. Add the vegetables, oil, herbs and jalapeño, if using. Mix well and season to taste with salt and pepper. *Serves 6.*

BARLEY BLACK BEAN SALAD

HIGHLY BENEFICIAL		NEUTRAL	O, A	AVOID	B, AB

This dramatic-looking salad tastes best when served at room temperature. Its medley of colors, textures, and flavors makes it an outstanding meal. You can serve it with a small wedge of either dairy or soy cheese and some homemade spelt bread.

½ cup dried black beans
1 tablespoon ground cumin
½ cup barley
3 ears fresh corn (TYPE O OMIT)
3 tablespoons chopped fresh coriander
½ red onion, chopped
¼ cup olive oil
lemon juice
salt

Soak black beans in water overnight; drain. Cover with fresh water. Add cumin and cook over low heat until tender, about 40 minutes. Drain, rinse well, and reserve in bowl. Boil barley until done, about 15 to 20 minutes. Drain, rinse, and add to black beans in bowl. Cut corn from cob and steam until tender; add to beans and barley. Mix in the coriander and red onion, then cover and chill mixture. Whisk olive oil, lemon juice, and salt to taste, and pour over salad. Toss ingredients together. This dish can be eaten at room temperature or served cold. *Serves 4.*

ADZUKI BEANS AND SWEET BROWN RICE

HIGHLY BENEFICIAL	O, A	NEUTRAL		AVOID	B, AB

For a mixed–blood type family, this bean and rice combination can be served as a main course, or as a side dish with grilled chicken or fish. Steamed broccoli or a mixed green salad completes the meal.

2 to 3 cups cooked adzuki beans (leftover or canned is fine)
2 cups sweet brown rice
4 cups water or vegetable stock
2 teaspoons salt
1 small red onion, diced small
¼ cup chopped fresh cilantro
2 oz. crumbled goat cheese

Adzuki are small and delicate, and really don't have to be soaked overnight. If you put them to soak in the morning, they'll be ready to cook by the afternoon. Cook the beans according to the package directions. Combine rice, stock or water, and salt in a 2-quart saucepan and bring to a boil. Reduce heat, cover, and simmer until done, about 35 to 40 minutes. If using canned (rinse first) or leftover beans, heat up. In a large serving bowl, combine the hot rice and beans, the onion, and the cilantro. Mix well, but gently. Top with crumbled goat cheese and serve. *Serves 4 to 6.*

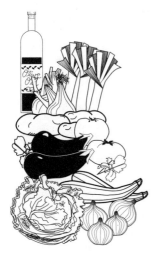

TWELVE

Vegetables

*T*HE FLAVORS AND TEXTURES OF MOST VEGETABLES are best expressed through simple treatment. Eaten raw, steamed, baked, or sautéed, vegetables should accompany every meal, the more the better.

The recipes that follow provide creative ways to prepare vegetables when you're looking for something different and interesting. Just remember: the simpler the preparation, the better.

GLAZED TURNIPS AND ONIONS

HIGHLY BENEFICIAL	O, A	NEUTRAL	B, AB	AVOID	

Turnips are an often overlooked vegetable choice. Cook them as you would carrots. Small turnips don't need to be peeled if they're fresh and unwaxed. Otherwise, peel the turnip and put in hot water 10 minutes. This makes them easier to digest and reduces their rather sharp, pungent odor. Highly Beneficial for Type O and Type A, they are of Neutral value to Type B and Type AB. Turnips are a terrific source of vitamin C, potassium, and folic acid. Turnip greens are rich in vitamins A, B, and C as well as potassium and magnesium. The greens can be cooked as you would spinach.

2 tablespoons butter (TYPE A USE OLIVE OIL)
2 tablespoons olive oil
1 yellow onion, quartered
4 turnips, cut into wedges
4 cloves garlic, crushed and peeled
¾ to 1 cup chicken stock (TYPE A AND TYPE AB USE WATER)
salt
3 to 4 tablespoons fresh parsley, chopped

In a heavy skillet, melt the butter in the oil over low heat. Add onion, turning to coat with butter and oil, and cook over very low heat until soft and deep golden in color, about 20 minutes. Add turnips and garlic, turning well. Add chicken stock or water and a little salt and bring to boil. Reduce heat, cover, and simmer until done, about 20 minutes. Check to be sure there is always liquid in the skillet. Add a few tablespoons at a time as needed. There should be very little liquid left. Remove lid and allow the last of the liquid to evaporate. Continue to turn vegetables. Serve at once, spooning sauce over them and sprinkling with parsley.   *Serves 4.*

CARROTS AND PARSNIPS WITH GARLIC, GINGER, AND CILANTRO

HIGHLY BENEFICIAL	O, A, B, AB	NEUTRAL		AVOID	

Carrots and parsnips, humble root vegetables that they are, reach new heights of gustatory delight when paired with garlic, ginger, and cilantro. The depth and sweetness of the carrot and the savory richness of the parsnip provide a wonderful complement to the sharp zing of the fresh ginger.

olive oil
2 carrots, sliced on the diagonal
2 parsnips, sliced on the diagonal
6 cloves garlic, crushed and peeled
½- to 1-inch piece of fresh ginger, minced
water
4 tablespoons fresh cilantro, chopped
salt

Heat 1 to 2 tablespoons oil in a heavy skillet over medium heat. Add vegetables, and turn in the oil a few moments until coated. Add garlic and ginger, stirring another moment. Add ½ cup water and bring to a boil. Reduce heat, cover, and braise 15 to 20 minutes, or until carrots and parsnips are tender. Be sure that there is always a little water in the skillet, adding a tablespoon or two as needed. As the dish nears completion, water should be absorbed. At the last moment of cooking, add the chopped cilantro and salt to taste.   *Serves 3 to 4.*

SWEET POTATO PANCAKES

HIGHLY BENEFICIAL	O, B, AB	NEUTRAL		AVOID	A

Sweet potatoes are a vitamin A–packed treat. They are lovely when baked, and are great in casseroles and stews. These pancakes are a perfect accompaniment to grilled meats and roasts, and are equally delicious with poultry and fish.

1 large sweet potato, or 4 cups grated
¼ red onion, grated
2 tablespoons chopped fresh cilantro
1 large egg
¼ cup spelt flour
¼ teaspoon salt
¼ cup olive or canola oil for cooking

Wash and rinse sweet potato; do not peel. Grate over a large plate. Add onion and cilantro. Mix in egg and flour until well incorporated, then add salt. The mixture will be loose, but will form patties. In a large skillet, heat oil and carefully pan-fry each cake 4 to 5 minutes on each side. Once cooked, the pancakes can be kept warm in a 250-degree F oven for an hour or so.

Makes 6 large dinner-size pancakes, or 15 appetizer-size pancakes.

CAULIFLOWER WITH GARLIC AND PARSLEY

HIGHLY BENEFICIAL	B, AB	NEUTRAL	AB	AVOID	O

Cauliflower is a densely packed flowering vegetable with a potent nutritional wallop. Its mild flavor is an excellent foil for many different flavors, in particular garlic, curry, and nutmeg. This is a Highly Beneficial vegetable for Type B and Type AB. While of Neutral value for Type A, its benefits make it a valuable addition to the diet. And don't forget the hybrid of broccoli and cauliflower, *broccoflower*, a pale green cruciferous vegetable loaded with nutritional goodness.

1 head cauliflower
2 tablespoons olive oil
4 to 6 cloves garlic, crushed and peeled
water
3 to 4 tablespoons chopped fresh parsley
salt

Cut cauliflower into fairly uniform sections. In a large, heavy skillet, heat 2 tablespoons oil. Add garlic, sautéeing until fragrant. Add cauliflower pieces and turn in the oil. Then add about a cup of water and bring to a low boil. Cover pan and let the cauliflower steam. When cauliflower is soft but firm, the water should be almost absorbed. If not, remove the lid and let most of the excess liquid boil away, leaving a rich oil and garlic sauce. With the back of a wooden spoon, coarsely mash cauliflower. Add parsley and salt to taste. Served with pan-roasted chicken or fish, this is also a satisfying pasta sauce.   *Serves 4.*

BRAISED FENNEL AND GARLIC

HIGHLY BENEFICIAL		NEUTRAL	O, A, B, AB	AVOID	

Fennel has a sweet, earthy flavor lightly tinged with anise that goes well with fish. This simple preparation seems well suited to this often overlooked but glorious vegetable.

1 bulb fennel
2 tablespoons olive oil

3 cloves garlic, crushed and peeled
water
½ teaspoon salt
3 to 4 tablespoons fresh parsley, chopped

Cut fennel into ¼-inch-thick slices, using as much of the fennel as possible. The stalks are a little fibrous, but can be saved for stock or used here. Heat oil in a heavy skillet over low to medium heat. Add sliced fennel and stir to coat with oil. Add garlic, ½ cup water, and salt and bring to a gentle simmer. Cover and cook until tender, 15 to 20 minutes. Be sure to keep a little water in the skillet, adding extra by the tablespoon as needed. During the last few minutes of cooking, add parsley.   *Serves 3 to 4.*

STEWED STRING BEANS WITH TOMATOES AND GARLIC

HIGHLY BENEFICIAL		NEUTRAL	O, AB	AVOID	A, B

This is a traditional Greek method of preparing string beans. The long, slow cooking in the acidic tomato and pungent garlic makes the beans tender. String beans are a Neutral value for all the blood types, and tomatoes are Neutral for Type O, so slide this dish to your side of the table and enjoy.

2 tablespoons olive oil
4 cloves garlic, chopped
1 to 1½ lbs. string beans, washed and stems removed
28 oz. can whole plum tomatoes
1 teaspoon dried oregano
salt

Heat oil in a casserole dish over medium heat. Add garlic and sauté briefly. Add beans and stir to coat with oil. Add the plum tomatoes, crushing them before they go into the pot. You can use a knife to coarsely chop them, or break them up by hand. Bring to a boil, and then reduce heat to a low simmer. Stir in oregano and a generous pinch of salt, cover, and cook mixture 45 minutes to 1 hour. The beans should be very tender and the tomato liquid almost absorbed. For the last several minutes of cooking, slide the lid aside so that most of the steam escapes, leaving a rich, thick sauce.   *Serves 4 to 6.*

MASHED PLANTAINS

HIGHLY BENEFICIAL		NEUTRAL	B, AB	AVOID	O, A

Plantains look a lot like bananas and are easy to find, usually in the tropical foods section of the produce aisle. They're of Neutral value to Type B and Type AB, but can be a welcome change from potatoes.

2 ripe plantains
1 tablespoon butter
1 tablespoon olive oil
salt

Peel plantains. Though similar in appearance to bananas, plantains don't peel like bananas. You'll probably have to cut them into smaller pieces first. After peeling, cut them into 1-inch thick slices and place in a pot. Cover them completely with water and bring to a boil. Cook until they are fully tender, 20 to 30 minutes. Keep an eye on them, because riper plantains will cook more quickly. Don't overcook. Drain, reserving a little of the broth. Mash well, adding butter and olive oil. Season with salt to taste. You may want to use the cooking water, a spoonful at a time, in the mashing process.   *Serves 3 to 4.*

BRAISED GREENS WITH GARLIC

HIGHLY BENEFICIAL	O, A, B, AB	NEUTRAL		AVOID	

There is a rich, nutritious world of mildly bitter to sharply bitter greens waiting to be discovered and cooked. Greens are easy to prepare, available year-round, and complement anything from grains to tofu, fish, meats, and poultry. And greens are compatible for all blood types. What better recommendation could they possibly have? The following recipe is a general guide for braising these great greens. Braising them slowly makes them easier to digest, and their nutrients are better assimilated in our bodies. The flavors vary tremendously, from mildly piquant to bitter, with a number of the greens having a hot, peppery bite. Recommended are chard, mustard greens, collards, kale, escarole, chicory, dandelion greens, broccoli rabe (sometimes sold as rappini), beet greens, and turnip greens.

1 bunch greens
2 tablespoons olive oil
4 to 6 cloves garlic, crushed and peeled
water
salt

Wash the greens very well, because some of them are exceptionally gritty, and carelessness at this stage of preparation can result in a less than pleasant dining experience. Some greens have leaves that are very wide. Cut them against the grain of the stems at 1-inch intervals into long strips, and don't discard the stems. Eat them, too. Heat oil in a heavy skillet with a lid over medium heat. Add garlic and sauté until it softens. Add cut green leaves, turning them in the oil. The leaves will be voluminous, but they will reduce in size substantially by the time they're ready to be eaten. Reduce heat and cook for several minutes. The moisture retained during washing should be all the water the greens initially need. After several minutes, add ½ cup water and cover skillet. Check frequently to be sure there is still water, adding a few tablespoons at a time as necessary. Doneness varies from green to green. They should be soft and limp, and most of the water should have evaporated. Add salt to taste.   *Serves 2 to 3.*

PURÉED CAULIFLOWER WITH PESTO

HIGHLY BENEFICIAL	B, AB	NEUTRAL	A	AVOID	O

The swirl of green pesto in this pure white purée is very pretty, and the taste is unusual.

1 head cauliflower
2 cloves garlic, crushed and peeled
salt
Basil Pesto (see page 324)

Quarter cauliflower, place in top of double boiler, and sprinkle with garlic. Pour boiling water over cauliflower and garlic and steam until cauliflower is soft enough to pierce with a straw, 15 to 20 minutes. Transfer to blender or food processor and purée until smooth. Add salt to taste. At the table, spoon a dollop of pesto onto each serving.   *Serves 4.*

PAN-FRIED SWEET POTATOES OR YAMS

HIGHLY BENEFICIAL	O, B, AB	NEUTRAL		AVOID	A

Yams and sweet potatoes have been confused with one another for so long that they've become one and the same tuber in many minds. Certainly, some yams and sweet potatoes are similar in appearance, but there are some two hundred varieties of yams and four hundred varieties of sweet potatoes! Yams are earthier tasting and less sweet than sweet potatoes. Baking sweet potatoes in their skins induces the flesh of certain varieties to yield a considerable amount of natural sugar. They can be quite good served this way, with perhaps a dab of butter. They are also a nutritious year-round treat, full of potassium, vitamin A, and vitamin C. Baked yams and sweet potatoes can be refrigerated and eaten cold as a healthy snack. While sweet potatoes are Highly Beneficial for Type O, Type B, and Type AB, sweet potatoes *and* yams are on the Avoid list for Type A. This recipe is quick and easy. So quick that you've got to keep a sharp eye on it so as not to scorch the slices. Allow one sweet potato or yam per person, depending on the size of the tuber.

yams or sweet potatoes
2 to 3 tablespoons olive oil per potato
salt

Preheat oven to 250 degrees F. If you prefer, peel yams or sweet potatoes, although the well-scrubbed skin is quite good. Slice them no thicker than ⅟₁₆ inch. In a large, heavy, preferably cast-iron skillet, heat oil over medium heat. Carefully add potato slices, fitting as many in the skillet as possible. Let them gently fry for a few minutes, occasionally lifting a slice to be sure it hasn't burned. There will be dark brown spots over the underside of the slices. Turn the slices at this point. Fry on the other side for a minute or two. Each slice should be soft (poke it with a fork). Transfer slices to plate. You can drain them on a towel if you'd like, although the olive oil tends to run off anyway. Sprinkle with a little salt and keep them warm in the oven while you repeat this process with the remaining slices. Keep an eye on the heat of the oil and the browning on the slices.

VEGETABLE FRITTERS

HIGHLY BENEFICIAL	O, A, B, AB	NEUTRAL		AVOID	

Fritters can be a light supper on their own or an excellent accompaniment to chicken or fish. Depending on your blood type, squash, sweet potatoes, yams, carrots, and turnips are all good choices for this fritter recipe. Grate the vegetables finely. If there's any excess liquid, drain and reserve before adding the rest of the ingredients.

3 cups grated vegetables
1 tablespoon finely minced onion
2 eggs
olive oil
salt

Mix grated vegetables with onion and eggs. The batter will be quite wet. In a large, heavy skillet, heat 3 tablespoons oil over medium heat. Lightly shape a handful of the batter for each fritter and gently drop into the oil, taking care not to splatter yourself. Flatten the fritters with a spatula. Let them brown over medium heat until the bottoms begin to color. Turn the fritters over and fry for several more minutes. Drain on paper towels, sprinkle with salt, and serve. You can also keep them warm in a preheated 250-degree F oven while you cook the rest of the batter. *Serves 4 to 6.*

STEAMED ARTICHOKE

HIGHLY BENEFICIAL	O, A	NEUTRAL		AVOID	B, AB

Everyone has developed their own approach to artichokes, and if it works for you, carry on. And remember: Although the meat at the bottom of the leaves contains small amounts of the very potent sugar produced in the artichoke heart, the prized and succulent heart itself is a treasure trove of potassium, magnesium, and folic acid. While artichokes are Highly Beneficial for Type O and Type A, they are on the Avoid list for Type B and Type AB. It pays to know your blood type!

1 stalk lemongrass, peeled and cut into pieces (large is okay)
1-inch piece fresh ginger, peeled and julienned
1 teaspoon olive oil
4 cloves garlic, crushed and peeled
1 artichoke per person

Place all ingredients in the steamer. With or without trimming, the stem left long or cut short, the bottom up or tips down, an artichoke usually takes between 45 and 55 minutes to thoroughly cook. Keep plenty of water in the bottom of the pan, and the pot mostly covered. Serve with a squeeze of lemon juice or a dipping sauce. Allow 1 artichoke per person.

SWISS CHARD WITH SARDINES

HIGHLY BENEFICIAL	O, A, B, AB	NEUTRAL		AVOID	

This recipe is suited to all of the blood types if the tomato is eliminated for Types A and B. Swiss chard is Highly Beneficial

for Types O and A, and is a Neutral value to Types B and AB, off-
set by the tremendous nutritional boost of the sardines, which
are loaded with calcium.

> *2 lbs. Swiss chard*
> *2 tablespoons olive oil*
> *3 cloves garlic, minced*
> *1 small onion, thinly sliced*
> *6 sardines, packed in water, drained and chopped*
> *1 tomato, chopped* (TYPES O AND AB)
> *salt*

Wash chard well, slice into 1-inch strips, and steam quickly. Remove from pan and set aside. In a large skillet, heat oil over
medium heat. Add garlic and onions and cook until slightly
browned and soft. Add sardines and tomato. Add greens and
toss lightly, cooking all ingredients together for a few more
minutes. Season with salt to taste.   *Serves 4.*

GARDEN RATATOUILLE

HIGHLY BENEFICIAL		NEUTRAL	O, A, B, AB	AVOID	

If you are lucky enough to have your own garden, or a generous
neighbor who does, this recipe will come in handy at the end of
the summer, when there is always an overabundance of green
and yellow squash, plum and cherry tomatoes, and basil. There
are no hard and fast rules here. If your vegetable bin yields a
mushroom or two, so much the better. Of course, choose only the
best vegetables for your blood type. The basic recipe is as simple
and elegant as the result is nutritious and delicious!

> *3 tablespoons olive oil*
> *1 medium onion, diced*
> *5 cloves garlic, chopped*

3 green zucchini (medium), sliced lengthwise,
then cut into chunks
3 yellow squash (medium), prepared as above
1 or 2 cups tomatoes, chopped, or cherry tomatoes, halved
(TYPE A AND B OMIT)
salt
½ cup fresh basil, chopped
grated pecorino romano cheese (optional)

In a large, heavy skillet, heat oil, add onion and cook 3 minutes, then add garlic and cook another 3 minutes. Add squash and cook, turning every 5 minutes, for 15 minutes. Type O and AB add tomatoes, reduce heat, and continue to cook another 10 minutes. Season with salt, toss with fresh basil, and top with grated cheese, if desired. Serve with rice or pasta as a main course, or with grilled meats, chicken, or fish.   *Serves 6.*

BRAISED COLLARDS

HIGHLY BENEFICIAL	O, A, B, AB NEUTRAL		AVOID	

Collard greens were traditionally cooked for hours with a piece of fatback bacon. For our purposes, however, a little olive oil replaces the bacon fat. Collard greens are not only delicious and nutritious, but Highly Beneficial for all of the blood types. Collards also are great as cold leftovers. You can use them as a filling for a frittata or an omelette. For Type O, Type B, or Type AB, there is no better way to fuel the body for a day's excursions than an omelet or frittata with leftover collards.

3 tablespoons olive oil
1 large onion, thinly sliced
1 large bunch fresh collard greens, washed well, tips of stems
removed (the stems are quite delicious)

2 tablespoons soy sauce or tamari sauce (optional)
small amount of water, as needed

Heat oil in a very large skillet or saucepan. Add onion and cook 5
minutes. Meanwhile, slice collards by rolling them into 1 large
bunch, then cutting across the leaves in 1-inch intervals. Wash
them, and with water on their leaves add all the collards to the
pot at once, cover, and reduce heat. After 5 minutes, turn the
collards so the wilted greens are on top. Add soy sauce or
tamari, if using, and replace cover. Cook another 40 minutes,
turning collards occasionally to make sure they cook evenly.
Add a tablespoon or two of water at a time, as needed. Unlike
other greens, collards are tastier if allowed to cook longer.
Serves 4.

GRILLED PORTOBELLO MUSHROOMS

HIGHLY BENEFICIAL		NEUTRAL	O, A, B, AB	AVOID	

These dense, meaty mushrooms are a great vegetarian substitute
for hamburgers. Try them with garlic over pasta, or serve them as
a satisfying and tasty side dish. Be sure to brush liberally with
garlic and olive oil.

4 large Portobello mushrooms, stems removed
(reserve for soups or stews)
4 teaspoons Garlic-Shallot Mixture (see page 334)
4 slices soy cheese (optional)
1 tablespoon olive oil
salt
chopped fresh parsley or basil
4 homemade spelt buns

Prepare grill. Brush mushrooms liberally with Garlic-Shallot Mixture, olive oil, and herbs. Grill over medium heat 5 to 8 minutes. Turn over. If using soy cheese to make cheeseburger substitutes, place cheese on top. Whether you use cheese or not, grill another 5 to 8 minutes. Season with salt, sprinkle with fresh herbs, and serve on homemade spelt buns. Or, serve with grilled meat, poultry, fish, tempeh, and a nutty brown rice. *Serves 4.*

BRAISED LEEKS

HIGHLY BENEFICIAL	O, A	NEUTRAL	B, AB	AVOID	

Leeks are Highly Beneficial for Type O and Type A, while of Neutral value to Type B and Type AB. Try braising them with other vegetables, or use them in soups, stews and casseroles.

1 large leek
2 cloves garlic, sliced
2 tablespoons olive oil
salt
½ cup water or vegetable stock

Wash leeks thoroughly, removing green tops and root ends; slice thinly. Heat oil in a heavy cast-iron skillet over medium heat. Add sliced garlic and sauté a few moments. Add leeks and stir to coat with oil and garlic. Cover pan and gently cook leeks, adding a tablespoon of water at a time, until they are soft and thoroughly cooked. Season with salt.   *Serves 3 to 4.*

GRILLED PEPPER MEDLEY

HIGHLY BENEFICIAL	B	NEUTRAL	O	AVOID	A, AB

Red peppers, orange peppers, yellow peppers, and green peppers; sweet peppers and hot peppers—there are few things more delicious than roasted or grilled peppers, or a sautéed mixture of peppers, onions, and tomatoes. Toss in some other Highly Beneficial vegetables. Hot peppers, in their multitude of varieties, belong in a category of their very own. One of the things we do know about peppers is that they're powerhouses of vitamin C; the more red the better.

3 peppers, mixed (sweet red, green, yellow, or orange)
1 large onion (white, yellow, Bermuda, Spanish, or Vidalia)
2 cloves garlic
2 tablespoons olive oil
2 tablespoons chopped fresh parsley
salt

Core and seed peppers; slice thinly. Chop over onion into small pieces. Crush garlic. Heat oil in a heavy cast-iron skillet over medium heat. Add garlic and onion and sauté gently until they become translucent. Add peppers and toss to coat them with oil. Sauté mixture until peppers are soft. Add chopped parsley and toss gently. Add salt to taste.   *Serves 4.*

THIRTEEN

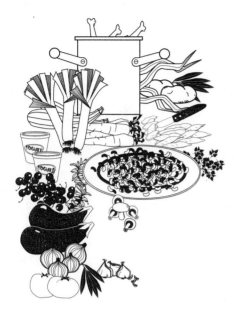

Soups & Stews

*S*OUPS AND STEWS HAVE SUSTAINED NATIONS. THE apocryphal story of rock soup isn't that far from the truth. Somehow, the concept of a communal pot into which any ingredient could be added became the metaphor for cultures and civilizations. Soups and stews are much the same, varying only in the proportion of broth to solid ingredients. They are filling and nutritious, providing a simple, one-pot, cook-ahead meal that often tastes even better on the second or third day. Soups and stews are avenues to dietary inspiration. The majority of refrigerators, pantries, and gardens contain ample ingredients for a soup. Frozen meat, fish, chicken, or vegetable stock; vegetables; beans; pasta; leftover meats, chicken, fish—the list of potential ingredients is endless. Soups and stews provide a terrific opportunity to use up leftovers and can be prepared in sufficient quantity to supply more than one meal.

The first two recipes that follow are for basic homemade stocks. These stocks are vastly superior to canned broths and bouillon cubes.

BASIC TURKEY STOCK

HIGHLY BENEFICIAL	AB	NEUTRAL	O, A, B	AVOID	

Homemade stocks frozen in individual batches provide a great head start for preparing any number of sumptuous dishes. A good stock is basic to any sauce, soup, or stew. Creating a stock really takes very little effort. There are a number of ways to approach it. For instance, you can roast a turkey and set aside the carcass, neck, and giblets for a stock. Or purchase necks and backs from the butcher, and use these as the basis for a hearty stock. Either of these methods will provide a tasty stock. Turkey is Neutral for Type O, Type A, and Type B, and Highly Beneficial for Type AB—a perfect stock for all blood types! Turkey, once considered only a holiday bird, is now available year-round. The ingredients should always be fresh. A turkey stock can also be enhanced by mushroom stems, herbs, onion peels, leek stalks, or celery leaves. Don't add vegetables such as broccoli, cauliflower, or Brussels sprouts; they are cruciferous vegetables which will add an unpleasantly sulphurous taste and odor to the stock.

1 medium turkey carcass, picked fairly clean
(reserve any leftover meat for soup)
2 onions, roots removed, skins on, and cut into quarters
3 large carrots, cut into chunks
3 stalks celery, washed and cut into large pieces
¼ bunch fresh parsley, including stems, washed
fresh herbs, such as thyme, rosemary, oregano, basil, to taste
bay leaf or sage

Fill a very large (5 to 6 quart) stock pot three-quarters full with water. Add all of the ingredients and bring to a boil. Reduce heat and simmer at least 2½ hours. The stock should reduce by a third. Let cool to room temperature, and skim any scum or fat from the surface. Refrigerate. Once cold, the fat will harden on top of the stock. At the same time, the scum will sink to the bottom. Stock made with bones will gel when cold. The stock can be frozen in convenient pint and quart containers. *Makes approximately 4 quarts.*

BASIC VEGETABLE STOCK

HIGHLY BENEFICIAL	O, A, B, AB NEUTRAL	AVOID

Vegetable stock is simmered only 40 minutes, unlike turkey stock which needs to cook slowly over many hours to develop its rich flavors. This vegetable stock is "sweet" and clean-tasting, and full of nutrients. Again, don't use the cruciferous vegetables broccoli, Brussels sprouts, or cauliflower; they will dominate the taste of the broth.

1 large yellow onion, cut into quarters
2 carrots, washed, trimmed, and cut into large pieces
2 stalks celery, washed and cut
parsley stems
garlic skins
apple skins and cores
mushroom stems
parsnips
leeks

Fill a very large (5 to 6 quart) stockpot three-quarters full with water and bring to a boil. Add all the vegetables and herbs and

simmer 40 minutes. Cool and strain out the vegetables. Refrigerate or freeze.   *Serves 4 to 6.*

APPLE-CURRY LAMB (LEFTOVER) STEW

HIGHLY BENEFICIAL	O, B, AB	NEUTRAL		AVOID	A

This dish uses the recipe for Grilled Curried Leg of Lamb (see
page 125).

¼ cup canola oil (TYPE B SUBSTITUTE OLIVE OIL)
2 medium apples, washed, quartered, cored, and cut into pieces
2 stalks celery, washed and sliced
1 large onion, peeled and diced
2 tablespoons ground curry powder
1 tablespoon ground cumin
½ teaspoon cayenne (TYPES O AND B ONLY)
2 tablespoons spelt flour
1 cup rice or almond milk
1 lb. cold cooked lamb, fat removed and cut into bite-size pieces
¼ cup raisins
salt

In a large skillet or heavy saucepan, heat oil over medium heat.
Add apples, celery, and onion, and cook until wilted. Add
spices and cook 2 minutes. Add flour and cook 5 more minutes. The mixture will be a bit sticky, but cook the flour as
long as possible, being careful not to scorch it. Add rice or almond milk, lamb, and raisins and stir well to combine. Let
simmer ½ hour, adding some water or chicken stock if sauce is
too thick. Add salt to taste. Serve with basmati rice, chutney,
and other condiments.   *Serves 3 to 4.*

🍴 CYBER RECIPE 🍴

ASIAN STEW

AUTHOR: Kay A (Alex1Kay@aol.com)

TYPE A

This is a homestyle soup that's also low in calories. It will keep for several days in the refrigerator and reheats well.

5 cups vegetable stock (Sometimes I substitute a bit of chicken stock.)
1 small onion, thinly sliced
2 cloves garlic, minced
1 tablespoon minced gingerroot
2 tablespoons soy sauce
3 stalks bok choy, sliced on diagonal with leaves shredded
1 cup broccoli florets
1 carrot, shredded
1 cup sliced Portobello mushrooms (or your favorite "A" mushroom)
½ cup shelled peas
1 cup water chestnuts, sliced
2 ounces buckwheat noodles or soba noodles, broken into 1-inch pieces (about ½ cup)
½ lb. firm tofu, cut into ½-inch cubes

Pour ½ cup of the stock in a 5-quart saucepan and bring to a boil. Add onion, garlic, and ginger and simmer 3 minutes. Stir in remaining stock and soy sauce. Cover pot and bring to a gentle boil. Add remaining ingredients as they are prepared. Test for doneness: Noodles should be softened; vegetables should remain crisp-tender. Timing: 8 to 10 minutes. *Serves 6.*

INDIAN LAMB STEW WITH SPINACH

HIGHLY BENEFICIAL	B	NEUTRAL		AVOID	O, A, AB

Buy a leg of lamb, cut it in half, and use part for this stew and the other half for shish kabobs. The meat for the stew should be cut into cubes smaller than those for the skewers. This is a good way to prepare two dinners at the same time.

3 tablespoons olive oil
1 large onion, chopped
2 tablespoons ground mustard
2 tablespoons ground cumin
2 tablespoons ground coriander
4-lb. leg of lamb, cut in half and cubed small
(reserve other half for kabobs)
1 cup plain yogurt (low-fat is good)
water
4 to 5 cloves garlic, peeled and diced
2-inch piece fresh ginger, peeled and diced
2 lbs. fresh spinach, cleaned and chopped
salt

In a large stew pot or saucepan, heat oil over medium heat. Add onion and cook several minutes, until translucent. Add all the spices and cook 2 to 3 minutes to release the flavors. Add lamb, mixing to coat well with the spices. Bit by bit, stir in yogurt and add enough water to cover. Stir in garlic and ginger and simmer meat, covered, until tender, about 1 hour and 15 minutes. Remove cover and simmer another 15 minutes, if necessary, to reduce liquid. Add spinach in batches, stirring it down to incorporate it into the stew. It will cook in just a few minutes. Season with salt to taste, and serve with saffron rice and mango chutney. (Type B only.) Like all other stews, this one can be made ahead and even frozen. It really does improve the second day. *Serves 4.*

VENISON STEW

HIGHLY BENEFICIAL	O, B	NEUTRAL		AVOID	A, AB

Venison has substantial nutritive value and almost no fat. Deer overpopulation has led to death by starvation for tens of thousands of these beautiful creatures. Selective hunting can not only feed the hungry, but also keep the deer population healthy. The venison available through specialty meat companies like D'Artagnan, is often farm-raised, so unlike its wild relative, it doesn't require extensive marinating to break down the fibrous muscle tissue. Still, its flavor is enhanced if you marinate it in wine for a day or so.

1 package (1¼ lbs. to 2½ lbs.) venison
1 fist-sized onion, cut into pieces
wine
5 juniper berries
2 bay leaves
2 tablespoons olive oil
1 onion, diced
2 carrots, peeled and sliced
1 small turnip, sliced
2 stalks celery, sliced
1 small parsnip, peeled and sliced
½ lb. mushrooms

The venison meat is usually cut into flank steaks, so you need to cut each of the steaks into bite-size pieces. Place in a ceramic bowl. Add onion and cover with wine. Add juniper berries and bay leaves, cover with plastic wrap, and refrigerate a day or two.

When you are ready to make the stew, strain and reserve wine; discard onion, juniper berries, and bay leaf. In a heavy casserole large enough to accommodate the meat, vegetables, and wine, heat over medium heat. Add diced onion and sauté until golden. Add venison and brown quickly, being careful not to crowd the pot or the meat will steam. Brown the meat in batches if necessary. Pour reserved wine over meat and bring to a boil. Reduce heat and simmer 45 minutes to 1 hour. Add carrots, turnip, celery, and parsnip. Continue to cook until vegetables are tender. Add mushrooms and cook a few more minutes until done.   *Serves 4 to 5.*

BEEF STEW WITH GREEN BEANS AND CARROTS

HIGHLY BENEFICIAL	O	NEUTRAL	B	AVOID	A, AB

The great thing about stews is that there are no hard and fast rules on the seasonings and various ingredients. If you have some mushrooms, throw them in at the last minute. (If they are dried, put them in with the carrots.) If you prefer thyme, oregano, and rosemary, use those herbs instead of the ground spices. Follow the parameters of the recipe and create your own version according to Blood Type. Replacing the beef with cubed lamb would make this a Highly Beneficial dish for Type O, Type B, and Type AB, if you omit the chili powder. The beef stew is only Highly Beneficial for Type O and is of Neutral benefit for Type B.

2 lbs. stew beef, cut into 1-inch cubes
¼ cup spelt flour (or less, for dredging meat)
3 tablespoons olive oil
1 tablespoon ground cumin
½ tablespoon ground kelp
1 tablespoon chili powder

1 teaspoon salt
⅓ cup red wine
2 to 3 cups stock (chicken, vegetable, or meat)
1 tablespoon Garlic-Shallot Mixture (see page 334) or
1 medium onion plus 2 cloves garlic, chopped
4 skinny carrots, peeled and sliced on the diagonal
1 lb. green beans

Cut away any fat from the meat. Dredge lightly in flour and shake off any excess. Heat oil in a large pot over moderate heat and brown beef in 2 batches. After the second batch is nearly done, return first batch of meat to the pot, then add all the spices and salt. Cook 5 minutes on low heat, then add wine to deglaze. Add 2 cups stock, then stir in shallot mixture. If using onions and garlic, add them. Cover pot and simmer 1 hour, checking periodically to see if more liquid is needed. Add if necessary. Add carrots, cover, and simmer another 30 minutes. Check for tenderness. Add green beans and cook another 10 to 15 minutes. Serve with buttered rice noodles or with rice and homemade bread. A terrific leftover.   *Serves 6.*

VEAL STEW WITH FENNEL

HIGHLY BENEFICIAL	O	NEUTRAL	B	AVOID	A, AB

Great fall flavors pervade this tender and savory stew. Fennel is a stalk vegetable with an appearance and texture similar to those of celery, but its flavor is reminiscent of mild licorice. Fennel has been used as a vegetable, an herb, and as a medicinal plant since ancient times. It is considered a diuretic, an antispasmodic, and a stimulant, able to soothe gastric distress, cleanse the system, and even prevent flatulence. As a vegetable, it can be eaten raw, lightly steamed, or braised. It combines nicely with onion and parsley.

2 lbs. veal, trimmed of fat and cubed
½ cup spelt flour
¼ cup olive oil
1 medium onion, diced
1 medium fennel bulb, sliced
3 tablespoons chopped, fresh parsley
1 teaspoon salt
¼ cup white wine
2½ to 3 cups stock (according to type)

Dredge veal in spelt flour. Shake off excess. In a large, heavy skillet, heat oil over medium heat and brown veal in several batches, turning once. Remove meat and reserve in a large stockpot. Once all the meat is browned and in the pot, sauté the onion and fennel together in the same skillet until golden. Add parsley and salt and mix well. Deglaze pan with wine and add everything to the stew pot. Add 2½ cups stock and bring just to a boil. Reduce heat, cover, and simmer 1½ hours. Be careful not to boil; the meat toughens.   *Serves 4.*

TURKEY SOUP

HIGHLY BENEFICIAL	AB	NEUTRAL	O, A, B	AVOID	

With a rich turkey stock waiting to be used, it only takes a few more ingredients to produce a satisfying and filling turkey soup—a classic comfort food at its best on cold fall or winter evenings.

8 cups turkey stock
2 carrots, diced small
2 stalks celery, diced small
1 scallion, sliced (optional)
1 cup turkey meat, torn into small pieces

1 cup noodles (rice or spelt)
1 tablespoon salt

In a large pan, bring stock to a near boil. Add carrots and celery and simmer about 20 minutes, or until vegetables are tender. Add scallion, turkey, and noodles, and simmer another 10 minutes, or until noodles are al dente. *Serves 4.*

GINGERED SQUASH SOUP

HIGHLY BENEFICIAL	O, A, B, AB	NEUTRAL		AVOID	

Any of the winter squashes can be used to produce this simple, zesty soup: Pumpkin, butternut, acorn, delicata, hubbard, or kabocha squashes are all quite delicious. The squashes range in color from a pale yellow to a deep orange. The use of a turkey stock enriches the flavor while contributing a protein boost.

1 large winter squash
4 cloves garlic, peeled
1-inch piece fresh ginger, chopped
1 teaspoon salt
3 cups water or turkey stock

Carefully peel squash. Most squash tend to be quite hard, so caution is advised in the initial preparation. Always cut flat side down. Cut squash in half and scoop out seeds. Seeds can be set aside for roasting, as they're not only delicious but also a valuable source of zinc. Continue to cut squash into smaller pieces until you have manageable cubes. Peel cubes with a small, sharp knife. Cut into pieces and place in a heavy-bottomed pot. Add garlic, ginger, and salt. Cover with water or turkey stock and bring to a boil. Reduce heat and simmer until the squash is tender and easily pierced with the tip of a knife. Transfer mixture to a food processor or blender and purée until smooth.   *Serves 4 to 6.*

MIXED ROOTS SOUP

HIGHLY BENEFICIAL	O,A	NEUTRAL	B, AB	AVOID	

Mixed root vegetables simmered in either water or turkey stock make a wonderfully hearty fall or winter soup. Served with a crusty spelt bread and a green salad, this becomes an easy and a filling supper. Choose from the vegetables listed in any combination that you prefer. Some of the root vegetables, such as carrots, add a subtle sweetness to the soup. Cut all vegetables into a roughly uniform size so that they will cook at the same rate. Grate a little cheese over each serving, if you like.

2 tablespoons olive oil
1 cup diced leek or onion
6 cloves garlic, crushed and peeled
1 cup diced turnips or rutabagas
1 cup diced carrots
1 cup diced parsnips
boiling water to cover (about 8 cups)
salt
bay leaf
handful of chopped fresh parsley

In a heavy casserole dish, heat oil over medium heat. Add onion or leek and garlic and sauté until fragrant, about 5 minutes. Add hardest vegetables (turnips) first and turn in oil a few minutes. Add carrots and parsnips, turning several minutes more. Pour enough boiling water over vegetables to cover them by an inch. Add salt and bay leaf, and simmer at least 45 minutes, or until vegetables are tender. The soup can be coarsely mashed in the pot using a potato masher, or it can be put through a blender or a food processor. Remove bay leaf before blending. Don't blend it too well; the chunky textures of the root vegetables are very satisfying. Sprinkle with parsley. *Serves 10 to 12.*

CHERYL'S MISO-VEGETABLE SOUP

HIGHLY BENEFICIAL	A	NEUTRAL	O	AVOID	B, AB

Cheryl Miller is a longtime patient, friend, and practitioner of the Blood Type Diet. She's a great cook who has perfected many simple and delicious meals. This soup is quick and satisfying.

1 tablespoon olive oil
1 large clove garlic, finely chopped
1 medium white onion, chopped into small pieces
1 stalk celery, cut on the diagonal into thin slices
3 cups of broccoli, cut into small pieces
4 cups boiling water
2 tablespoons light miso
2 tablespoons tahini
salt and pepper

In a medium soup pot, heat olive oil, garlic, onion, and celery over medium heat, stirring until onion is slightly soft. Add broccoli and stir about 2 more minutes, until broccoli starts to wilt. Add 2 cups boiling water and the miso; stir well. Add remaining 2 cups water and bring to a boil. Boil 1 minute. If you have a portable mixer and can blend in the pan, add the tahini. Otherwise, remove half of the soup at a time and process with the tahini until smooth and creamy. Season with salt and pepper, if desired, and serve immediately.
Serves 6 to 8.

FRESH CHERRY AND YOGURT SOUP

HIGHLY BENEFICIAL	B, AB	NEUTRAL	A	AVOID	O

This is a classic summer soup to serve for a light breakfast or lunch. It can be served with a dessert bread, such as banana (Type B) or lemon (Type A, Type AB), a few slivers of goat or soy cheese, and a bunch of grapes.

1 lb. pitted cherries
3 tablespoons sugar
3 (2-inch) slivers orange peel (TYPES A AND AB SHOULD SUBSTITUTE LEMON PEEL)
2 cloves
3 cups water
2 cups yogurt
1 bunch fresh mint for garnish

Combine cherries, sugar, orange or lemon peel, and cloves with water and bring to a simmer. Poach gently until fruit is tender, 8 to 10 minutes. Remove cloves and coarsely mash cherries in the soup. Let cool. Add yogurt, mix well, and garnish with mint leaves.   *Serves 8.*

CREAM OF LIMA BEAN SOUP

HIGHLY BENEFICIAL		NEUTRAL	B	AVOID	O, A, AB

This creamy pale green soup is filling and provides a modest amount of protein. Serve with delicious homemade bread and some goat cheese. This is a quick version of the recipe. Instead of using dried lima beans that require long soaking, use frozen ones or fresh, if you can find them.

1 tablespoon butter
1 small onion, minced
2 cups low-fat milk
2 cups fresh, 1 package frozen, or 1 can drained lima beans
salt
3 tablespoons chopped fresh parsley for garnish

In nonreactive saucepan, heat butter over low heat. Add onion and sauté until soft. Add milk and beans and bring to a boil. Reduce heat and simmer gently until beans are tender. If using fresh or frozen limas, simmer 5 to 7 minutes. When beans are done, purée the milk and beans in a blender until smooth. Season to taste with salt. Garnish with chopped parsley. *Serves 4 to 6.*

CURRIED RED LENTIL SOUP

HIGHLY BENEFICIAL	A	NEUTRAL	AB	AVOID	O, B

Lentils aren't really legumes. They are pulses, the edible seeds of leguminous plants that originated in the Middle East. Lentils have been cultivated for over nine thousand years. At various times in their long history, lentils have been dismissed as the food of the poor. No matter. They've nourished countless civilizations and are intrinsic to many today. The largest consumer of lentils is India, where dozens of varieties are grown. We are most familiar with the brown, red, and green lentils. They are mildly flavored, which makes them adaptable to a number of different approaches. The beautiful orange of the red lentils, unfortunately, isn't retained once they are cooked. The good news is that, unlike beans, lentils don't require any presoaking, so this soup can be prepared within thirty to forty minutes. Pick through all lentils prior to cooking, watching carefully for tiny stones. Serve with braised greens and rice.

2 tablespoons olive oil
½ large onion, chopped
6 cloves garlic, chopped
2 tablespoons mild curry powder, or to taste
2 teaspoons cumin seeds
5 to 6 cups water
1½ cups red lentils, cleaned and rinsed
1 teaspoon salt
½ cup chopped fresh cilantro

In a heavy, lidded soup pot, heat oil over medium heat. Add onion and garlic, and stir for a few moments. Add curry powder and cumin and stir for a few minutes to fry the spices. The vegetables should be a lovely gold. Add water and bring to a boil. Stir in lentils. When water returns to a boil, reduce heat, partially cover, and simmer 15 to 20 minutes, or until lentils are soft. Add salt once lentils are done. Before serving, sprinkle with cilantro.   *Serves 6 to 8.*

MISO SOUP

HIGHLY BENEFICIAL	A, AB	NEUTRAL	O	AVOID	B

Miso, a fermented soybean paste, is a staple of Japanese cuisine. It ranges dramatically in color and flavor from light to dark, sweet to quite salty. Miso comes in so many varieties that it's best to see what's available and experiment. Some misos have rice, barley, and wheat added to them, so check the labels. Miso can be the base for soup or salad dressings. A light, delicious soup can be prepared in minutes if you have the stock ready. Traditionally, miso soup is prepared with bonito and kelp. Dried bonito isn't always easy to come by, but kelp can be found in health-food stores. The recipe here isn't truly authentic, because it's not based on dried bonito, but it would be a shame not to try this wonderful food for lack of a single ingredient. Trefoil, related to parsley and similar in appearance to cilantro, is another traditional ingredient. Trefoil isn't always easy to find, so try finely minced celery leaves, a few parsley leaves, or any other subtly flavored herb that appeals to you.

1 piece (about 8 to 10 inches) giant kelp (kombu), wiped
quickly with a damp cloth
1 quart water
4 tablespoons miso
½ cake tofu, cut into ½-inch cubes
additional vegetables, such as scallions, thinly sliced
mushrooms, tender dandelion leaves, celery leaves, light
green spinach leaves, and dried seaweed

Place kelp and water in a large bowl and let stand overnight. In the morning, discard kelp and pour liquid into a pot. Bring kelp stock to a simmer. Put miso in a bowl and add a few tablespoons of kelp stock, stirring to soften and blend the miso. Return the softened miso to the pot and return mixture to a low simmer. Add tofu and any other vegetables. Simmer briefly and serve with rice and salted cucumber slices.

There is a quicker, although more temperamental, version of the stock preparation: Place kombu and water in pot and bring just to a boil, *slowly.* Don't let the water boil, or the stock will be ruined. Pull out the kombu. If it's soft, the stock is ready. If the kelp is still too firm, return it to the pot and cook another minute or two. Again, do *not* boil. Add a few tablespoons of cold water over the brief cooking time. Once the stock is prepared, proceed as previously suggested. *Serves 4 to 6.*

CUCUMBER YOGURT SOUP

HIGHLY BENEFICIAL	B, AB	NEUTRAL	A	AVOID	O

This light, refreshing soup makes a simple, healthy lunch on a hot summer's day. Allow one cup of yogurt and one cucumber for every two servings.

1 cucumber
1 cup yogurt
squeeze of lemon
pinch of salt
½ cup fresh dill for garnish

If the cucumber skin isn't too tough or covered with a preserving wax, leave it on. Dice cucumber and put it in the blender with the yogurt, dill, lemon, and salt. Blend until almost smooth. Pour into a serving bowl and garnish with some fresh dill. If it's too thick, thin with water to desired consistency.
Serves 2.

ADZUKI BEAN & PUMPKIN SOUP
OR NAVY BEAN SOUP

HIGHLY BENEFICIAL	O, A, B, AB	NEUTRAL		AVOID	

This delicious soup is Highly Beneficial for Type O and Type A, if you use pumpkin, and the same for B and AB if you replace adzuki beans with navy beans.

2 tablespoons olive oil
2 medium leeks, washed well and thinly sliced
6 large cloves garlic, chopped

6 cups water
1 small (6 to 8 inches across) sugar pumpkin or 1 acorn or
butternut squash, peeled and cut into ½-inch pieces
1 can adzuki beans, drained and rinsed well
generous handful chopped parsley
salt

In a heavy pot, heat oil over medium heat. Add leeks and garlic
and turn to coat with oil. Cook a few minutes, until they begin
to color. Add enough water to cover them and bring to a boil.
Reduce heat and simmer 10 minutes. Meanwhile, prepare
squash. Add squash to pot, cover with water, and bring to a
boil. Reduce heat and simmer 15 to 20 minutes, depending on
variety of squash, or until tender. Stir in drained beans and
heat through. Add parsley for the last minute or two of cooking. Add salt to taste.   *Serves 4 to 6.*

HEARTY FISH SOUP

HIGHLY BENEFICIAL	O, A, B, AB	NEUTRAL		AVOID	

Fish soup can make an elegant and special meal. Each of the
blood types should choose a fish that is Highly Beneficial. Monkfish proves fine for everyone, so it can be used for a mixed–blood
type family. Combinations of various fish also make for a hardy
soup. Cod, snapper, grouper, and hake are just a few examples of
excellent soup fish.

2 tablespoons olive oil
1 small leek, finely sliced
6 to 8 cloves garlic, crushed and peeled
7 to 8 cups water
½ large parsnip, diced small
1 medium yellow pepper, diced small (Types O and B only)

1 to 1½ lbs. fish, cut into ½-inch pieces
1 to 2 cups tender, young leaves from celery,
or any greens, finely slivered
1 yellow tomato, chopped (TYPE O AND TYPE AB ONLY)
½ cup chopped parsley
salt

In a large soup pot, heat oil over medium heat. Add leek and sauté a few minutes. Add garlic and continue to cook another moment or two, being careful not to let the garlic burn, which turns it bitter. Pour in water and bring to a boil. Add parsnips and simmer 5 minutes. Add peppers and simmer 5 to 8 minutes. Add fish and return soup to a boil. Reduce heat at once. Add greens and tomato, then simmer 5 to 8 minutes longer, or until the fish is cooked. Stir in parsley and salt to taste. Serve at once. *Serves 4.*

WHITE BEAN AND WILTED GREENS SOUP

HIGHLY BENEFICIAL		NEUTRAL	O, A, B, AB	AVOID

This is an easy soup to make, and it's a great mixed–blood type pleaser. The cannellini beans are Neutral for all blood types. The Swiss chard is Neutral as well. As a colorful bonus, the chard tints the white cannellini beans a light pink.

1 can cooked cannellini beans, drained and rinsed
1 clove garlic, peeled and end trimmed
1½ to 2 cups stock or water
1 cup chopped Swiss chard
½ teaspoon salt

In a 2-quart saucepan, bring beans, garlic, and stock to a boil. Reduce heat and simmer 10 to 15 minutes. With a slotted spoon, scoop out beans and transfer to a food processor or blender with ½ cup of liquid. If you have one of those handheld blenders, leave soup in the saucepan and purée until smooth. Return purée to saucepan and stir until blended. Add greens, season with salt, and cook another 5 minutes. *Serves 2.*

CREAM OF WALNUT SOUP

HIGHLY BENEFICIAL	O, AB	NEUTRAL	A, B	AVOID	

2 cloves garlic, peeled and end trimmed
1½ cups walnuts
3 cups homemade turkey stock
½ cup dry white wine
½ cup soy, rice, or almond milk
salt and pepper
3 scallions, thinly sliced

Purée garlic in a food processor. Add walnuts and, while adding 2 cups of turkey stock, grind the nuts. Pour mixture into saucepan with remaining cup of stock. Add wine and soy milk and heat through. Season to taste with salt and pepper. Sprinkle with scallions before serving. *Serves 4 to 6.*

MUSHROOM-BARLEY SOUP WITH SPINACH

HIGHLY BENEFICIAL		NEUTRAL	O, A, AB	AVOID	B

The flavor and textures of this classic soup are extremely satisfying. The slightly honeyed essence of the barley and its smooth texture contrasts nicely with the mushroom and spinach. The spinach is best when fresh and added to the soup at the last minute, so it's still green and only slightly wilted.

1 tablespoon olive oil
1 small onion, diced
½ cup barley (uncooked)
1 tablespoon sherry
1 Portobello mushroom, halved and sliced
8 cups liquid, either turkey or vegetable stock (water is
acceptable, but the flavor will not be as rich)
1 teaspoon salt
2 cups fresh spinach, washed and stems cut or chopped

In a large pot, heat oil over medium heat. Add onion and cook 2 minutes, or until onion is wilted. Add uncooked barley, stirring until it is incorporated, and cook 2 minutes. Stir in sherry and mushroom. Cover, reduce heat, and simmer 2 minutes. When mushrooms have softened, add stock and bring to a boil. Reduce heat and simmer 45 to 50 minutes. Season with salt and add spinach. It will wilt very quickly.   *Serves 4.*

CURRIED CARROT SOUP

HIGHLY BENEFICIAL	A, B	NEUTRAL	O, AB	AVOID

This soup has eye-pleasing color, and the addition of the curry provides a spicy taste that contrasts wonderfully with the slightly sweet carrots.

½ stick butter (TYPE B) or canola-oil margarine (TYPE A)
or 3 tablespoons olive oil
1 large onion, peeled and diced
2-inch piece fresh ginger, peeled and grated
1 tablespoon curry powder
3 cloves garlic, crushed and peeled
2 lbs. carrots, washed and trimmed

1 cup dry white wine (optional)
7 cups chicken, turkey, or vegetable stock
1 sweet potato, peeled (TYPES O, B, AB ONLY)
salt and pepper

In a large pot, melt butter or margarine or heat oil over low heat. Add onion, ginger, curry, and garlic and cook until onions are translucent. Coarsely cut carrots and add with sweet potato to stockpot. Add wine and cook 1 minute, or until all the alcohol burns off. Add stock and simmer 45 minutes. Let cool slightly. Transfer mixture in batches to a food processor and purée. Return mixture to pot and season with salt and pepper to taste. If soup is too thin, reduce by simmering another 10 minutes, or until desired consistency is achieved.   *Serves 10 to 12.*

WILD RICE AND MUSHROOM SOUP

HIGHLY BENEFICIAL	A	NEUTRAL	O	AVOID	B, AB

This soup combines the taste of deep, earthy, wild mushrooms with the intense flavors of the dark, nutty-textured wild rice

2 cups wild mushrooms (abalone, Portobello, or tree oyster) or
4 oz. dried, reconstituted
6 tablespoons butter (TYPE O) *or canola-oil margarine* (TYPE A)
or 4 tablespoons olive oil
2 leeks, washed well and finely chopped
¼ cup minced garlic
⅓ cup spelt flour
8 cups chicken stock
½ cup dry white wine (optional)
1 cup wild rice
4 cups water for cooking rice

¼ cup sherry (optional)
sprig fresh thyme
salt

If using dried mushrooms, soak in water until soft. Drain, reserving soaking liquid, and chop mushrooms. In a soup pot, melt butter or canola-oil margarine, or heat olive oil. Add leeks and garlic, and sauté 1 minute. Add mushrooms and cook another 2 minutes. Add flour all at once and cook, stirring well, 2 minutes. Meanwhile, warm chicken stock and add 2 cups at a time to pot, whisking to incorporate. Add wine, if using. This is a basic gravy or roux, which is used to thicken sauces. Try to do this step slowly and in stages to avoid lumps. Simmer 1 hour. Separately boil the wild rice in plenty of water and drain while still al dente. Add rice to the simmering soup and cook 30 minutes longer. Add sherry, if using, and thyme, and cook 5 more minutes. Season with salt.
Serves 8 to 10.

CUBAN BLACK BEAN SOUP

HIGHLY BENEFICIAL	A	NEUTRAL	O	AVOID	B, AB

This is a thick and lemony bean soup that may be served either hot or cold. It becomes slightly grayish-purple with the addition of the lemon. Garnish by placing a slice of lemon on top of each serving. It's acceptable to use canned beans, and doing so makes for a really fast soup.

½ lb. dried black beans or 2 cans beans, drained and rinsed
1 onion, peeled and chopped
4 cloves garlic, crushed and peeled
4 to 5 cups chicken or vegetable stock
juice of 2 lemons, or ¼ cup juice

2 teaspoons salt
lemon slices for garnish or plain yogurt (TYPE A ONLY)

Wash and soak dried beans in three times the amount of water needed to cover and refrigerate overnight or for at least 8 hours. Drain and rinse beans. Combine beans, onion, garlic, and stock in large pot. Cook beans slowly over low heat until very tender, about 1 hour. Let cool slightly, then transfer to a food processor and purée in batches, adding liquid from pot to obtain desired consistency. Stir in lemon juice and salt. Serve immediately with a slice of lemon on top, or chill and serve with a dollop of plain yogurt (Type A only).   *Serves 6 to 8.*

WHITE GAZPACHO

HIGHLY BENEFICIAL	B, AB	NEUTRAL	A	AVOID	O

This is a wonderful variation of the classic tomato-based cold soup for those sweltering nights when one's appetite has been dimmed by the dog days of summer.

3 cucumbers, peeled and seeded
2 green peppers, washed and seeded (TYPE A AND AB OMIT)
1 red onion, cut in quarters
2 cups plain, organic yogurt
1 cup green grapes, coarsely chopped
vegetable stock as needed
2 tablespoons chopped fresh cilantro
2 tablespoons chopped fresh mint
salt

Cut cucumbers, peppers, and red onion into medium-size pieces. Combine them in a food processor and pulse on and off until they're not quite puréed. The texture should remain a bit chunky. Transfer to a large mixing bowl and whisk in yogurt. Thin as desired with vegetable stock or water with a little bit of white grape juice. Stir in the fresh herbs and grapes, and season with salt to taste.   *Serves 6 to 8.*

SIMPLE FISH SOUP

HIGHLY BENEFICIAL	A, B, AB	NEUTRAL	O	AVOID	

Exactly as its name describes it, this soup is simple. It can be served either hot or cold with a tossed green salad, crusty home-made spelt bread, and cheese—if it's permitted on your Blood Type Diet.

1 tablespoon olive oil
1 carrot, diced small
2 small stalks celery, diced small
½ onion, diced small
1 tablespoon sherry (optional)
4 cups water
¾ lb. grouper, cut into 1-inch pieces
2 tablespoons chopped fresh parsley

Heat oil in a saucepan over medium heat. Add carrot, celery, and onion and sauté several minutes. Add water. Add sherry, if using, and cook until vegetables are soft, about 10 minutes. Add grouper and simmer a few minutes longer, until the fish is thoroughly cooked. Sprinkle parsley over each serving.
Serves 2.

FOURTEEN

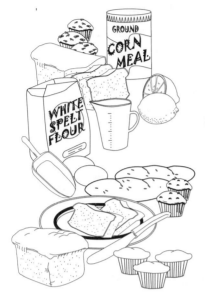

Breads, Muffins, Tea Cakes & Batters

HIS CHAPTER COVERS A WIDE VARIETY OF BAKED
goods. Bread baking is both an art and a science, but it is an art
that anyone can learn, and making your own bread is very rewarding. Children love to bake bread because it is a tactile, interesting experience, and they get to eat the results! The many
steps to traditional bread baking are all quite simple. They take
time, attention, and patience. Since time is not always something
we have, included here are recipes for bread machines as well.
The bread produced by a bread machine can't match the quality
of a hand-kneaded bread, but it's still very good, particularly if
the bread is going to be used for sandwiches.

There are also many delicious breads available commercially.
Most natural breads can be found in a health-food store, but carefully check the listed ingredients. Increasingly, commercial bak-

eries are using clever packaging to make their breads seem more wholesome, but refined wheat flour is still often the main ingredient. Essene and Ezekiel are the two commercial loaves that we highly recommend, but breads made with spelt, rice, and rye flours are also becoming more widely available.

To be a successful bread baker, it is important to remember these key points: Read the directions for the recipe before you start to bake. Always have the ingredients at room temperature. Try to be as precise in measuring all of the ingredients as possible. Make sure that your oven's temperature is correct. A variation of as little as twenty-five degrees can impact the baking process. The exciting news is that your baking skills will improve with each loaf of bread you make.

Hand-Kneaded Breads

FRENCH BREAD

HIGHLY BENEFICIAL	AB	NEUTRAL	O, A, B	AVOID	

1¼ cups warm water
¼ teaspoon sugar
1½ teaspoons active dry yeast
4 to 5 cups spelt flour (4 cups white spelt flour,
1 cup whole-grain spelt)
½ teaspoon salt
2 tablespoons cornmeal or rice flour
(if necessary, for baking sheet only)
egg wash (1 beaten egg)

Combine water, sugar, and yeast in a large mixing bowl. Stir until dissolved and let set 10 minutes. Add 4 cups white spelt flour and salt. Mix well with a dough hook attachment on a mixing machine or with a wooden spoon. When the dough is well mixed and still sticky, turn it onto a well-floured surface. Begin to knead by hand, adding in more flour (whole grain) as needed. Knead 10 minutes, or until dough is smooth and elastic. Put the dough in an oiled bowl, turn once to cover with oil, and cover with a clean dish towel. Place in a warm spot in your kitchen and let rise 2 hours. The back of the stove with a pilot light is ideal. Near a radiator or a warm stove is also good.

When the dough has doubled in size, punch down and divide in half. Roll into baguettes by folding the dough into itself, then rolling it with your hands from the middle outward. Place in French-bread pans, or place on a baking sheet dusted with cornmeal or rice flour. Brush each loaf with egg wash, cut 3 diagonal gashes about ¼ inch deep, and let rise a second time, about 30 minutes.

Preheat oven to 375 degrees F and bake loaves 30 to 35 minutes. Bread should sound hollow when tapped on the underside. *Yields 2 loaves.*

Note: To double this recipe, you may find that it only takes 7½ to 8 cups of flour. You can also substitute half whole-grain spelt and half white spelt flour for a denser, coarser texture.

RAISIN-PUMPERNICKEL BREAD

HIGHLY BENEFICIAL	AB	NEUTRAL	A, O	AVOID	B

A dark, flavorful loaf full of moist, sweet raisins. Delicious still warm out of the oven. Also delicious toasted.

½ tablespoon (1½ teaspoons) dry yeast, or ½ package yeast
1½ cups lukewarm water
½ cup molasses
1 tablespoon strong coffee, or 2 teaspoons
instant coffee (TYPE O OMIT)
1 tablespoon salt

2 cups rye flour
2 cups whole-grain spelt flour
2 cups white spelt flour
2 tablespoons canola oil
1 cup raisins
¼ cup cornmeal or rye cracker crumbs (for pan only)

Dissolve yeast in a bowl with lukewarm water. Let sit 5 minutes, then add molasses, coffee, and salt, and stir well. Add 5 cups flour all at once, and mix well with a heavy spoon. Turn onto a well-floured surface and knead in remaining 1 cup flour 8 to 10 minutes. Rye-flour breads tend to be a little stickier and take longer to rise than lighter doughs. Place in an oiled bowl, turn over once, and cover with a clean dish towel. Place in a warm area of the kitchen, allowing the dough to rise until three times its original size. It will take approximately 2 hours.

Turn dough onto a floured surface, and fold in the raisins by kneading the dough once more. Return to bowl, cover, and let rise again, but only until doubled. It will take approximately 30 to 40 minutes for this second rising.

Turn dough onto a floured surface and cut into thirds. Shape into three loaves or make small breakfast rolls. Dust baking sheet with cornmeal (or rye cracker crumbs) and set loaves apart from one another, leaving enough room for each loaf to rise. Cover until doubled in size.

Preheat oven to 375 degrees F and bake 35 to 40 minutes for bread, 20 to 25 minutes for rolls. Let cool on a rack.
Yields 3 loaves or 18 rolls.

QUINOA-FLOUR TORTILLA

HIGHLY BENEFICIAL		NEUTRAL	O, A, B, AB	AVOID	

Tortilla are a cooking staple rooted in pre-Hispanic Native American cooking. Tortillas are quickly prepared unleavened breads that are employed as the base for every meal. Quinoa flour is coarse like corn flour, or *masa harina*, so these tortillas are close in taste and texture to corn tortillas.

When you prepare tortillas, you'll understand and appreciate why village women have traditionally gotten together to make large batches of them. The ingredients are simple, and so is the procedure, but making tortillas is labor intensive. Share this endeavor with a friend or your child, because while one is rolling out dough, the other can be cooking them. It's a terrific way for friends to spend a couple of hours together and then enjoy the fruits of their labors. Serve with beans and a crisp romaine. Should there be any leftovers, slice into triangles, brush with olive oil, and bake in a preheated 350-degree F oven 10 minutes on each side. These make homemade tortilla quinoa chips and provide healthy little snacks for kids. You can also freeze the tortillas. To reheat, just toast on an open flame or in a preheated skillet, toss in a hot oven, or heat 15 seconds in the microwave.

2½ cups quinoa flour
1½ cups white spelt flour
1 teaspoon salt
1½ teaspoons baking powder
4 tablespoons canola oil
(TYPE B SHOULD SUBSTITUTE OLIVE OIL)
1½ cups warm water

In a large mixing bowl, combine dry ingredients and stir to blend. Add oil and water. Using a wooden spoon, mix until dough forms a ball. Turn onto a well-floured surface and knead 10 minutes. Cover loosely with plastic wrap, and let dough rest for 10 minutes. Divide dough into 14 pieces and form into balls. With a rolling pin, flatten each ball into a 10-inch tortilla. In a dry 12-inch skillet or griddle, cook each tortilla 1 minute on each side. Be sure not to overcook, or the tortillas will become too brittle. As you remove the tortillas from the pan, wrap in a large clean dish towel.   *Yields 14 tortillas.*

ENGLISH MUFFINS OR HAMBURGER ROLLS

HIGHLY BENEFICIAL		NEUTRAL	O, A, B, AB	AVOID	

You can sprinkle any beneficial seed over the tops of these little rolls: poppy, sesame, black sesame, or caraway. You can freeze what isn't consumed in the first serving. Toasted or grilled, used for burgers, dinner rolls, or sandwiches, these provide a tasty alternative to commercially prepared goods.

1 tablespoon active dry yeast
2 cups warm water
2½ teaspoons salt
5 to 5½ cups white spelt flour
¼ cup cornmeal, rye cracker crumbs, or rice flour
(for bottom of pan only)
egg wash (made from 1 beaten egg)
1 to 2 tablespoons blood type–specific seeds,
(optional)

Dissolve yeast in warm water and let sit 5 minutes. Add salt and most of the flour, reserving about ½ cup as needed. Mix well either by hand or with a dough hook until dough is manageable and can be turned onto a well-floured surface. Knead 8 to 10 minutes, incorporating the last ½ cup flour. Oil a large bowl, place dough in bowl, and turn once to coat with oil. Cover with a clean cloth and place in a warm area of your kitchen. Let rise until double in size. Turn dough onto a lightly floured surface and shape into 16 rolls. Pat down to flatten, then push with all your fingers away from the center and around the edges, as if you were preparing pizza. Place on a cookie sheet that has been sprinkled with cornmeal, rye cracker crumbs, or rice flour, leaving plenty of room between the rolls, because they'll rise again. Brush with egg wash, and top with seeds or leave plain. Most seeds are better toasted first. Preheat oven to 375 degrees. Cover rolls and let them rise once again, about 30 minutes. Bake 12 to 15 minutes, and let cool in pan. *Yields 16 rolls.*

WHOLE-SPELT SANDWICH OR HOT DOG ROLLS

HIGHLY BENEFICIAL	AB	NEUTRAL	O, A, B	AVOID	

1½ cups warm water
¼ cup soy powder
⅓ cup canola oil (TYPE B SHOULD SUBSTITUTE OLIVE OIL)
1½ teaspoons salt
1 tablespoon turbinado sugar
2 tablespoons active dry yeast
3 cups white spelt flour
2 cups whole-spelt flour
egg wash (egg beaten with 1 tablespoon water)
poppy or sesame seeds

Combine water, soy powder, oil, salt, and sugar in a mixing bowl. Stir to blend. Sprinkle yeast over this mixture and allow to dissolve a few minutes. Add 4 cups flour, reserving the last cup for kneading. Let rest for a minute, then knead 10 minutes. Oil a large mixing bowl, place dough in bowl, and turn once to coat with oil. Cover with a clean dish towel and let rise in a warm corner of the kitchen about 45 to 55 minutes, or until doubled in size.

Oil a sheet pan. Punch down the dough and separate into 2 pieces. With the first piece, squeeze into 8 rolls. Move them back and forth, from one hand to another, along a somewhat sticky surface, forming them into smooth rolls. With the other half, you can shape 6 to 8 cylindrical hot dog rolls. Brush with egg wash and sprinkle with poppy or sesame seeds (as allowed by blood type). Let rise again until doubled, about 45 minutes. Preheat oven to 425 degrees F and bake 20 minutes. Let cool on a rack. These little rolls freeze well.   *Yields 6 to 8 rolls.*

Bread Machines

THERE HAS BEEN a huge surge in the sale of bread machines in the last few years. They certainly take all of the hard kneading work out of the bread-baking process. The bread rises and bakes in the same pan the ingredients are mixed in! Pay careful attention to the measuring of ingredients: Too much or too little flour or water can have a direct impact on the taste and texture of your breads. Bread machines are designed to be used with specially milled flours, which are generally highly refined white or whole wheat. These have a higher gluten content than spelt flour, and so there are certain procedures that need to be changed when using the bread machine. The "mix" and "knead" settings tend to overmix the less glutinous spelt flour, so dissolve the yeast in the water rather than making it the last ingredient placed on top of the flour. Use the shortest baking cycle. For most bread machines, that would be the basic white-bread setting. Don't worry if you have to feed a loaf or two of bread to the birds, or turn it into bread pudding, before you get the taste and texture exactly the way you want them to be. Homemade bread, even using these incredibly convenient machines, is delicious, satisfying, and nutritious. Best of all, you can tailor these breads specifically for your blood type!

> ### Bread Machine Tip
>
> For more variety and a crustier consistency, set your machine on "dough," and bake the dough in the oven after it rises. You'll still save time and effort in the preparation.

PUMPERNICKEL BREAD

HIGHLY BENEFICIAL		NEUTRAL	O, A, AB	AVOID	B

This recipe makes a two-pound loaf of dark pumpernickel bread, with a strong and complex taste.

1⅔ cups water
1¼ teaspoons yeast
3 tablespoons soy powder
2 tablespoons canola oil
1 tablespoon honey
2 tablespoons molasses
2 teaspoons salt
1 cup whole-grain spelt flour
2⅔ cups white spelt flour
⅔ cup rye flour
2 tablespoons cocoa
2 teaspoons strong black coffee (TYPE O OMIT)

Measure all ingredients in the order listed into the bread machine's baking pan. Place in machine chamber, secure, and close lid. Select "whole-grain" setting and bake. Cool before slicing. *Makes 1 (2-lb.) loaf.*

HERB BREAD

HIGHLY BENEFICIAL	AB	NEUTRAL	O, A, B	AVOID	B

You can use whatever herbs you prefer. Rosemary, dill, marjoram, and basil all are well-suited to this bread. This recipe yields a hearty and interesting loaf of bread. Drizzle with olive oil and a little garlic before eating.

1½ cups water
1¼ teaspoons yeast
3 tablespoons soy powder
2 tablespoons canola oil
(TYPE B SHOULD SUBSTITUTE OLIVE OIL)
1 teaspoon turbinado sugar
1½ teaspoons salt
4 cups white spelt flour or, for whole grain, 3 cups white
spelt flour and 1 cup whole-grain spelt flour
1 to 2 teaspoons dried basil
1 to 2 teaspoons dried thyme

Measure all ingredients in the order listed into the bread machine's baking pan. Place in machine chamber, secure, and close lid. Select "basic white-bread" setting and bake. Cool before slicing.   *Makes 1 (2-lb.) loaf.*

WHOLE-SPELT BREAD

HIGHLY BENEFICIAL		NEUTRAL	O, A, B, AB	AVOID	

Spelt is different from its cousin wheat in many ways. When you eat spelt bread, you know the difference immediately. Spelt flour doesn't rise as much as refined white flour does. Instead, it makes a dense and slightly sweet loaf of bread with very satisfying taste and texture.

1 ½ cups water
1 ½ teaspoons yeast
2 tablespoons soy powder
2 tablespoons canola oil
(TYPE B SHOULD SUBSTITUTE OLIVE OIL)
2 tablespoons honey
2 tablespoons molasses
1 ½ teaspoons salt
3 ⅓ cups whole-spelt flour

Measure all ingredients in the order listed into bread machine's baking pan. Place in machine chamber, secure, and close lid. Select "white bread" setting and bake. Cool before slicing.
Note: For a slightly lighter loaf, substitute 1 cup of white spelt flour for 1 cup whole-grain spelt.   *Makes 1 (2-lb.) loaf.*

SPELT BREAD

HIGHLY BENEFICIAL		NEUTRAL	O, A, B, AB	AVOID	

This recipe makes ideal bread for sandwiches. For the lightest possible bread, use all-white spelt flour. But half whole grain and half white makes a chewy loaf that is a little higher in fiber than all-white spelt.

1 ½ cups water
1 ⅓ teaspoons yeast
2 tablespoons powdered soy milk
2 tablespoons canola oil
(TYPE B SHOULD SUBSTITUTE LIGHT OLIVE OIL)

2 teaspoons turbinado sugar
1½ teaspoons salt
2¼ cups whole-grain spelt flour
2 cups white spelt flour

Measure all ingredients in the order listed into bread machine's baking pan. Place in machine chamber, secure, and close lid. Select "basic" bread setting and whatever type crust desired, and bake. Cool thoroughly before slicing.
Makes 1 (2-lb.) loaf.

CINNAMON-RAISIN BREAD

HIGHLY BENEFICIAL		NEUTRAL	O, A, B, AB	AVOID	

1⅓ cups water
1¼ teaspoons yeast
2 tablespoons soy powder
2 tablespoons canola oil
(TYPE B SUBSTITUTE LIGHT OLIVE OIL)
1½ tablespoons turbinado sugar
1½ teaspoons salt
3 cups white spelt flour
1¼ cups whole-spelt flour
1½ teaspoons ground cinnamon
(TYPE O AND TYPE B SHOULD SUBSTITUTE NUTMEG)
1 cup raisins

Measure all ingredients, except raisins, in the order listed into bread machine's baking pan. Place in machine chamber, secure, and close lid. Choose "basic" setting and "regular" crust. When machine indicates, add raisins. Cool thoroughly before slicing.   *Makes 1 (2-lb.) loaf*

Muffins and Tea Cakes

MUFFINS AND TEA CAKES take only a few moments to prepare, cook fairly quickly, freeze well, and come in dozens of variations. They can make a healthy snack for children, are a perfect breakfast, or a satisfying little meal with a cup of green tea and a piece of fruit. Muffin and tea cake batters are raised with baking powder and baking soda. Unlike yeast-raised doughs, they don't need to rise before baking. They also require much less handling, so the lighter the touch the better. Texture is dramatically affected by *overmixing* these batters.

A plethora of dried and fresh fruits, as well as nuts and seeds, can make endless combinations in these sweet breads. Feel free to substitute other fruits, nuts, and seeds, according to your blood type.

BANANA-WALNUT BREAD OR MUFFINS

HIGHLY BENEFICIAL		NEUTRAL	O, B	AVOID	A, AB

The bananas make this bread sweet and moist, and the walnuts create an interesting counterpoint to the banana flavor.

oil for pans
2 cups white spelt flour
1 teaspoon salt
2 teaspoons baking soda
⅔ cup canola oil (TYPE B USE BUTTER)
1 cup turbinado sugar
1½ cups ripe banana chunks (about 2 large bananas)
3 eggs, beaten
½ cup chopped walnuts

Preheat oven to 350 degrees F. Prepare pans. If nonstick they don't need greasing; otherwise oil and flour the pans. If you're making muffins, you can use paper liners. Mix all dry ingredients in one bowl and all wet ingredients in another. Blend together and add walnuts for the last few turns with the spoon. *Don't overmix the batter.* Fill prepared pans three-quarters full, and bake 25 to 30 minutes for muffins, 30 to 35 minutes for prepared breads, or until a cake tester comes out clean. Let cool on rack. This is a great breakfast treat.

Note: For a whole-grain banana bread, substitute 1 cup whole-spelt flour for 1 cup white spelt flour.

Makes 1 dozen muffins or 3 small loaves.

BLUEBERRY MUFFINS

HIGHLY BENEFICIAL	A	NEUTRAL	O, B, AB	AVOID	

These muffins are both beautiful and dramatic. If you use buckwheat, they're dark and dense. But with any flour, the muffins take on a deep purple hue from the berries. They aren't too sweet and are great with a complementary all-fruit preserve.

oil or paper liners for muffin tins
1 cup buckwheat flour (TYPE O AND TYPE A)
1 cup oat flour (TYPE B AND TYPE AB)
1 cup white spelt flour
2½ teaspoons baking powder
½ teaspoon salt
⅓ cup sugar
2 tablespoons honey
1 cup soy milk
¼ cup canola oil (TYPE B SHOULD SUBSTITUTE BUTTER)
1 egg, beaten
½ cup blueberries, fresh or frozen

Preheat oven to 350 degrees F. Grease muffin tins or use paper liners. In a large bowl, mix dry ingredients together. In another bowl, stir together the honey, soy milk, oil, and egg. Lightly combine the dry and wet ingredients. Fold in blueberries. Fill each muffin cup to top. Bake 20 minutes, or until a toothpick comes out clean. *Makes 12 muffins.*

CORN BREAD

HIGHLY BENEFICIAL		NEUTRAL	A	AVOID	O, B, AB

Corn bread is a favorite accompaniment with soups and stews, as well as meat and bean dishes.

grease for pan
¾ cup white spelt flour
¾ cup stone-ground cornmeal
½ cup buckwheat flour
2 tablespoons brown sugar
2½ teaspoons baking powder
pinch salt
2 eggs
4 tablespoons canola-oil margarine, melted
1 cup soy milk

Grease a 9-inch square pan or cast-iron skillet and preheat in 425-degree F oven. Mix spelt flour, cornmeal, buckwheat flour, brown sugar, baking powder, and salt in one bowl. In another bowl, beat eggs well. Add melted margarine and soy milk and stir until blended. Add liquid ingredients to dry, stirring quickly until just mixed. *Do not overmix.* Pour into hot pan or skillet and bake 20 to 25 minutes. Serve hot. *Makes 12 pieces.*

QUINOA-ALMOND MUFFINS

HIGHLY BENEFICIAL			NEUTRAL	O, A, B, AB	AVOID	

These are moist and full of the unique flavor of quinoa, which has a light, almost hazelnut, taste to it.

butter, oil, or paper liners for pan
1 cup quinoa flour
1 cup white spelt flour
⅓ cup turbinado sugar
2½ teaspoons baking powder
¼ teaspoon salt
1 egg
1 cup soy or rice milk
½ cup canola oil (TYPE B SHOULD SUBSTITUTE
LIGHT OLIVE OIL OR BUTTER)

Preheat oven to 400 degrees F. Prepare muffin tins using butter, oil, or paper liners. In one bowl, combine all dry ingredients. In another bowl, beat egg. Add almond milk and oil and stir until blended. Add liquid ingredients to dry, stirring quickly until just mixed. Fill tins to almost full. Add water to remaining empty tins, and bake 15 to 20 minutes. *Makes 12 muffins.*

BANANA-PLUM BREAD

HIGHLY BENEFICIAL	B	NEUTRAL	O	AVOID	A, AB

Serve this moist, not-too-sweet loaf for breakfast. Type Bs can try spreading it with a little sweetened ricotta, while Type Os can use fresh goat cheese. Add the larger amount of nuts and lemon rind if you prefer. Type O can use all-spelt flour.

butter for pans
1 cup spelt flour
¾ cup oat flour
2½ teaspoons baking powder
½ teaspoon salt
5 tablespoons softened butter
⅔ cup turbinado sugar
1 to 2 teaspoons grated lemon rind
1 to 2 eggs, beaten
1 cup mashed banana
3 ripe plums, diced
½ to 1 cup walnuts, broken into pieces

Preheat oven to 350 degrees F. Liberally butter two 8½ × 4½ × 2-inch loaf pans. Sift flours, baking powder, and salt into one bowl. In another bowl, blend butter, sugar, and lemon rind until creamy. Beat in eggs and mashed banana. Add dry ingredients to butter mixture in 3 parts, beating well after each addition. Fold in plums and walnuts. Pour into prepared loaf pans. Bake about 40 minutes, or until a straw comes out clean. Cool. This slices well. *Makes 2 small loaves.*

LEMON TEA CAKE

HIGHLY BENEFICIAL		NEUTRAL	O, B	AVOID	A, AB

With the addition of the lemon glaze, this cake stays moist for several days. Refrigerate to retard spoilage.

¾ cup butter, at room temperature
¾ cup turbinado sugar

3 eggs, beaten
1 tablespoon lemon juice
zest of same lemon
1½ cups white spelt flour
¾ teaspoon baking powder
¼ teaspoon salt

LEMON GLAZE

1 cup water
juice of 2 lemons
¼ cup honey

Preheat oven to 350 degrees F. Butter and flour two 8½ × 4½ × 2-inch loaf pans. In a mixing bowl, blend butter and sugar until light and fluffy. Add eggs, lemon juice, and zest (the outer, colored portion of the lemon). Gradually add flour, baking powder, and salt, scraping down the sides of the bowl. *Do not overmix.* Fill prepared pans to almost three-quarters full, and bake 25 minutes.

Meanwhile, prepare glaze: Combine all ingredients in a small saucepan and simmer about 10 minutes. The glaze should be thick but still pourable. While cake is still warm, pour glaze over top, allowing it to run down sides. Let cool.

PUMPKIN-ALMOND BREAD

HIGHLY BENEFICIAL		NEUTRAL	O, A, AB	AVOID	B

A moist, sweet, slightly spicy tea bread with an interesting texture, thanks to the ground almonds.

butter or oil for pan
1 cup white spelt flour

¾ cup ground almonds
½ teaspoon baking powder
1 teaspoon baking soda
½ teaspoon salt
½ teaspoon cinnamon (TYPES A AND AB)
⅛ teaspoon cloves
⅛ teaspoon nutmeg (TYPE O OMIT)
½ teaspoon ginger
¾ cup turbinado sugar
¼ cup butter, at room temperature (TYPE O ONLY; TYPE A AND
TYPE AB MAY SUBSTITUTE CANOLA-OIL MARGARINE)
2 eggs
1 cup pumpkin
⅓ cup soy milk
½ cup raisins or chopped figs

Preheat oven to 350 degrees F. Grease a 9 × 13-inch glass pan. In
a large bowl, mix flour, ground almonds, baking powder, baking soda, salt, cinnamon, cloves, nutmeg, and ginger. In a separate bowl, beat the sugar, butter or margarine, and eggs until
very light. Add pumpkin and beat again. Swiftly add dry ingredients alternately with soy milk in two additions. Stir in
raisins or figs. Pour into prepared pan and bake about 30 minutes, or until a straw comes out clean.   *Yield: 1 loaf*

Batters for Pancakes and Waffles

PANCAKES AND WAFFLES don't have to be weekend luxuries. They
don't even have to be eaten for breakfast. If you keep a mixture
of the dry ingredients in a container, all you have to do to enjoy
these filling pancakes or dessert crêpes is to heat the griddle or
waffle iron, add the wet ingredients, and pour the batter.

BARLEY AND SPELT PANCAKES

HIGHLY BENEFICIAL		NEUTRAL	O, A, AB	AVOID	B

1 cup barley flour
1 cup spelt flour
2 teaspoons baking powder
pinch of salt
2 eggs
1½ cups soy milk
water as needed
butter, margarine, or oil for skillet

Combine flours, baking powder, and salt in a large bowl. Stir well to combine. In a separate bowl, beat eggs very well and stir in soy milk. Pour liquid into dry ingredients and stir until blended. The addition of water here depends on whether you prefer thick or thin pancakes. Heat butter, margarine, or oil in a heavy skillet. When hot, ladle in batter. Cook on low heat until bubbles fully cover the surface of the pancakes. Turn over and cook until beautifully colored. Serve with maple syrup, honey, or your favorite all-fruit preserves.
Makes 15 to 20 medium-size pancakes.

MILLET, SPELT, AND SOY PANCAKES

HIGHLY BENEFICIAL	B, A, AB	NEUTRAL	O	AVOID	

1 cup millet flour
½ cup spelt flour
½ cup soy flour
1 tablespoon baking powder
pinch of salt

2 eggs
1½ to 2 cups soy milk
water as needed
butter, margarine, or oil for skillet

Combine flours, baking powder, and salt in a large bowl. Stir well
to combine. In a separate bowl, beat eggs and add soy milk,
mixing well. Pour liquid into dry ingredients and blend thoroughly. Heat butter, margarine, or oil in a heavy skillet. When
hot, ladle in batter. Cook over low heat until bubbles fully
cover surface of pancakes. Flip over and cook until lightly colored on underside. Serve with maple syrup, honey, or your favorite all-fruit preserves. *Makes 15 to 20 pancakes.*

AMARANTH PANCAKES

HIGHLY BENEFICIAL		NEUTRAL	A, AB	AVOID	O, B

Served with honey, maple syrup, or just fresh fruit, these pancakes are full of the exceptional protein, vitamins, and minerals
that amaranth can provide. Amaranth contains twice the iron and
four times the calcium of wheat—an excellent way to provide
nutritious fuel for the day's labors.

1 cup amaranth flour
1 cup white spelt flour
1 teaspoon sugar
½ teaspoon salt
1 teaspoon baking powder
2 eggs, beaten
1 cup low-fat ricotta cheese
1 cup water
½ teaspoon almond extract
butter, margarine, or oil for skillet

In a medium bowl, mix flours, sugar, salt, and baking powder. Stir
well to combine. In another bowl, blend eggs, ricotta, water,
and almond extract. Pour liquid into dry ingredients and
blend without overmixing. The batter may seem a bit thin,
but after sitting 5 minutes it thickens. Heat butter, margarine,
or oil in a heavy skillet. When hot, spoon in batter. Cook over
medium heat until bubbles form on surface. Turn over and
cook until lightly colored.   *Makes 15 to 20 pancakes.*

BROWN RICE AND SPELT PANCAKES

HIGHLY BENEFICIAL	B, AB	NEUTRAL	O, A	AVOID	

These are delicious pancakes, and the combination of whole-
spelt and brown rice flours gives them a lot of natural sweetness
and body. They are spectacular with fresh berries. Type Bs be
sure to check the label on your rice milk. Some brands use canola
oil.

1 cup brown rice flour
1 cup whole-spelt flour
1 teaspoon baking powder
2 eggs
1½ cups rice milk
butter, margarine, or oil for skillet

In a medium bowl, combine flours and baking powder, mixing
well. Beat in eggs and rice milk. Heat butter, margarine, or oil
in a heavy skillet. When hot, ladle in batter. Cook over
medium low heat until bubbles appear on the surface. Flip
over and cook until lightly browned. Serve with maple syrup,
honey, or a favorite all-fruit preserve.
Makes 15 to 20 medium-size pancakes.

FIFTEEN

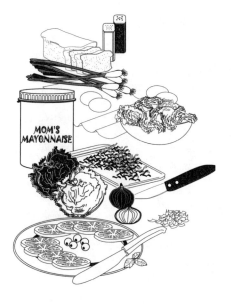

Salads

*E*ACH OF THE BLOOD TYPES HAS A TASTY VARIETY OF
vegetables to choose from. Blood types are limited only by the
vegetables that have been indicated as Avoid on their individual
lists. Even though many vegetables are listed as of Neutral value
for a specific type, the tastes, textures, and valuable nutrients
should be enjoyed anyway for their aesthetic and food value.

COLE SLAW

HIGHLY BENEFICIAL	B	NEUTRAL	AB	AVOID	O, A

This colorful version of the American classic has more bite and crunch than its simpler predecessor.

½ head white cabbage
¼ head red cabbage
½ head Chinese cabbage
2 carrots, grated
1 red onion, chopped
¾ to 1 cup homemade mayonnaise (see page 318)
2 tablespoons horseradish
½ teaspoon celery salt
1 teaspoon caraway seeds
¾ to 1 cup walnuts, broken into pieces

Finely sliver the leaves of all 3 cabbages to make 6 to 8 cups. In a large bowl, combine cabbage with grated carrots and chopped onion and toss until well mixed. Combine mayonnaise, horseradish, celery salt, and caraway seeds in a small bowl. Pour dressing over cabbage leaves and toss to combine. Let marinate in the refrigerator several hours to develop flavors. Add walnuts just before serving. *Serves 6 to 8.*

MESCLUN SALAD

HIGHLY BENEFICIAL		NEUTRAL	O, A, B, AB	AVOID	

Mesclun is a salad of mixed greens that was difficult to find in any but the finest gourmet restaurants until a couple of years ago.

Mesclun is readily available in the markets now. Even organic mesclun is widely available. There are varied mixtures, but certain lettuces are inevitably part of the ingredients: Swiss chard and spinach are standard greens, as are frisée, red- and oak-leaf lettuces, radicchio, arugula, and watercress. The slightly peppery arugula and watercress contrast nicely with the colorful, crunchy radicchio, and the entire salad is quite pretty. A fresh white apple sliced over the top with a drizzle of olive oil and a squeeze of lemon make a lovely presentation.

1 lb. mesclun greens
*2 medium tomatoes, sliced (*Type O and Type AB only*)*
1 cucumber, peeled and sliced
¼ cup crumbled feta or mild goat cheese
Olive Oil & Lemon Dressing (see page 326)

Spoon 2 tablespoons of dressing into a large bowl. Add the mesclun. Toss with another tablespoon of the dressing so there's a light coating on the greens. Top with sliced tomato and/or cucumber and crumbled feta or goat cheese.
Makes 4 large salads.

SPINACH SALAD WITH EGG & BACON

HIGHLY BENEFICIAL	O, A	NEUTRAL	B, AB	AVOID	

Fresh is best, but wilted spinach with a warmed vinaigrette is also very pleasing.

1 lb. fresh spinach
Olive Oil & Lemon Dressing (see page 326)
1 hard-boiled egg, chopped
2 slices organic turkey bacon, cooked and chopped
2 tablespoons grated romano cheese
salt

Wash the spinach several times to clean it of dirt and grit. Remove tough stems. Pat or spin dry. Place in a large salad bowl. Heat dressing and pour it over the spinach. Toss well to mix. If not wilted enough, then put spinach and dressing back into the pan for a minute. Top with chopped egg, turkey bacon, and grated cheese. Add salt to taste.   *Serves 2.*

GREEK SALAD

HIGHLY BENEFICIAL	O, A	NEUTRAL	B, AB	AVOID	

Certain ingredients need to be toyed with and others omitted from this all-time favorite, but the basic flavors remain the same. The romaine lettuce is highly beneficial to Type O and Type A, and of Neutral value to Type B and Type AB, which makes it fine for all.

⅓ cup Olive Oil & Lemon Dressing (see page 326)
1 tablespoon fresh mint, chopped
2 tablespoons fresh basil, chopped
2 tablespoons fresh parsley, chopped
2 cucumbers, washed, peeled and sliced
1 green pepper, halved, seeded, and cut into bite-size pieces
(Type A and Type AB omit)
2 stalks celery, chopped
1 small red onion, sliced
1 clove garlic, diced
1 head crisp romaine, washed, dried, and torn into
bite-size pieces
¼ cup crumbled Greek feta cheese
Greek olives (Type AB only)
1 teaspoon fresh or dried oregano

In a large salad bowl, mix the dressing, the herbs, and all of the vegetables. Reserve the romaine, cheese, and olives. Cover vegetables and marinate in refrigerator 1 to 2 hours. Toss the romaine with the marinated vegetables. Top with the crumbled feta and the olives. Sprinkle with a dusting of oregano. Mix well. *Serves 2 to 4.*

MIXED MUSHROOM SALAD

HIGHLY BENEFICIAL		NEUTRAL	O, A, B, AB	AVOID	

This salad is often found as an antipasto in Italian restaurants. However, it's also delightful as a side dish served on a bed of shredded romaine.

10 to 12 oz. mushrooms, according to blood type
1 cup vinaigrette
2 tablespoons chopped fresh parsley
2 tablespoons chopped fresh chives
2 cups shredded lettuce

Choose a salad dressing for your blood type. For many, the Sweet Vidalia Onion Dressing (page 327) or oil and lemon will serve nicely. Marinate mushrooms in 1 cup dressing for 1 or 2 hours. Mix in fresh herbs. Divide lettuce among 4 salad plates. Using a slotted spoon, drain mushrooms and serve over lettuce. *Serves 4.*

CARROT-RAISIN SALAD

HIGHLY BENEFICIAL	A, B	NEUTRAL	O, AB	AVOID	

This updated classic provides a sweet, crunchy accompaniment to almost any light summer meal.

2 lbs. carrots, washed, trimmed, and grated
½ cup raisins, plumped in hot water
3 tablespoons mayonnaise (TYPE A SUBSTITUTE
OLIVE OIL AND LEMON DRESSING)
3 tablespoons chopped fresh Italian parsley or
chopped fresh cilantro
1 scallion, thinly sliced, or 1 tablespoon chopped fresh chives

Place carrots in a serving bowl. Drain the raisins and mix with the
carrots. Add remaining ingredients and toss well.   *Serves 4.*

GRILLED SWEET-POTATO SALAD

HIGHLY BENEFICIAL	O, B, AB	NEUTRAL		AVOID	A

This is a very refreshing side dish that makes great use of extra
cooked sweet potatoes

2 lbs. sweet potatoes, sliced raw and then grilled
3 tablespoons olive oil
1 scallion, sliced
2 tablespoons chopped fresh parsley
2 tablespoons chopped fresh cilantro
juice of 1 lime

Cube the sweet potatoes after they've cooled. If you can refrigerate them for a while, they'll taste even better. In a large bowl,
combine sweet potatoes with remaining ingredients, toss well,
and serve. *Serves 4 to 6.*

ALDER-SMOKED MACKEREL SALAD

HIGHLY BENEFICIAL		NEUTRAL	O, A, B, AB	AVOID	

This works for lunch or hors d'oeuvre on rye or rice crackers. However, smoked fish should be eaten rarely and only if you have no digestive problems. Try it as a filling for scooped-out cherry tomatoes for Type O and Type AB. Put a half-spoonful on cucumber slices or at the base of small endive leaves.

4 smoked mackerel fillets, skinned and boned
½ red onion, diced small
⅓ to ½ cup Olive-Oil Mayonnaise (see page 318)
juice of 1 lemon

Chop fillets by hand. Combine fillets and remaining ingredients in small bowl. Mix well and serve with crackers.
Yields approximately 2 cups.

COLD GRILLED CHICKEN SALAD

HIGHLY BENEFICIAL		NEUTRAL	O, A	AVOID	B, AB

Grill chicken parts on hot grill, turning to cook each side, about 40 minutes. After chicken parts have finished grilling, set them aside and let them cool. Remove skin, take meat from the bone, and slice into smaller pieces until you have between one and two cups. White breast meat is the least fatty of chicken parts.

1 to 2 cups diced chicken
3 tablespoons Olive-Oil Mayonnaise (see page 318)
juice of 1 lime

3 tablespoons chopped fresh cilantro
2 scallions, thinly sliced
1 red pepper, either roasted or grilled, with skin removed
or fresh, cut in half, then sliced (TYPE O ONLY)
salt

Put the prepared chicken in a bowl. Thin mayonnaise with lime juice and add to chicken. Add remaining ingredients, toss well, and serve with crackers, on Ezekiel bread, or rolled in a romaine leaf.   *Serves 2 to 4.*

GREAT CAESAR SALAD

HIGHLY BENEFICIAL		NEUTRAL	O, A, B, AB	AVOID	

Romaine is such a sturdy lettuce that it naturally complements a strong and textured dressing. If you don't want to use anchovies, kelp will make a flavorful and nutritious substitute, while preserving the essence of the original salad. The dressing can stand alone as a dip for fresh vegetables or tempeh. The croutons should be made from stale spelt bread. The best croutons are made from French-style bread.

THE SALAD

1 head romaine, washed and dried
4 anchovy fillets, drained and set aside

THE DRESSING

1½ tablespoons Olive-Oil Mayonnaise (see page 318)
juice of 2 lemons
1 cup extra-virgin olive oil

2 tablespoons kelp powder
5 large cloves garlic
¼ cup grated pecorino romano cheese

Prepare dressing: Spoon mayonnaise into a mixing bowl. Without washing the food processor, blend lemon juice, olive oil, kelp, garlic, and cheese into a paste. If it gets lumpy and needs thinning, then add 2 tablespoons of the mayonnaise, and blend until smooth. Combine the two mixtures by hand for a pungent and delicious dressing.

THE CROUTONS

¼ cup olive oil or canola oil
2 cloves garlic, put through a press
1 tablespoon salt
2 cups cubed stale bread, according to type

Prepare croutons: Preheat oven to 425 degrees F. In a small bowl, combine oil, garlic, and salt and whisk until blended. Add cubed bread and toss to coat with the mixture. Place cubes on a cookie sheet with plenty of room between them for toasting and bake 5 minutes. Turn and bake another 2 to 4 minutes, or until golden brown. Remove from oven and cool thoroughly. Croutons may be stored in an airtight container for several days, though they're better when used immediately.

Prepare salad: Tear or cut the leaves of romaine. In a large bowl, toss romaine with the dressing. Top with croutons and four strips of anchovy. (Type O only.) Serve chilled.   *Serves 4.*

GREEN BEANS, CHÈVRE, AND WALNUTS

HIGHLY BENEFICIAL	O, A	NEUTRAL	B, AB	AVOID	

This is simple to prepare and great for entertaining. The green beans are Highly Beneficial for Type A and the walnuts are Highly Beneficial for Type O, but all blood types can enjoy this dish. This dish is best served at room temperature, but during the warmer summer months you may want to chill it first.

2 lbs. green beans, stems removed
¼ cup walnut pieces and halves
2 tablespoons crumbled goat cheese
2 tablespoons extra-virgin olive oil
squeeze of lemon juice
salt

Quickly blanch the green beans by throwing them into a pot of boiling water and counting to a slow 30. Then transfer them to an ice bath. Drain well and dry. On a serving plate, layer the beans, walnuts, and crumbled goat cheese. Dress with good olive oil and a squeeze of lemon juice. Add salt to taste. *Serves 4 to 6.*

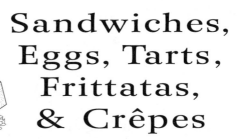

Sandwiches,
Eggs, Tarts,
Frittatas,
& Crêpes

ERE ARE A WIDE RANGE OF SIMPLE, INEXPENSIVE recipes that provide wonderful ways to use leftovers. You can also use whatever you happen to have in your vegetable bin or pantry. A few staples can form the basis for a satisfying and quick supper, or for an elegant meal for unexpected company. It's a good idea to have the fundamentals for these recipes on hand: A loaf of fresh or frozen bread, eggs, a couple of cheeses, pasta, olive oil, a jar or two of preserves, nut butters, sardines, tuna, fresh vegetables, and a pot or two of fresh herbs gracing your window. Dried herbs are just fine, though.

Leftovers are the key to many of the recipes offered in this chapter, and there's no better way to plan ahead than when the grill or oven is already heated up for some other meal. Pull whatever you have out of the vegetable bin—carrots, onions, sweet potatoes, mushrooms, leeks, tempeh, tofu, apples—cut into pieces, brush with olive oil, sprinkle with salt, and grill or broil, five minutes on each side. Let cool, refrigerate, and in the next day or two, incorporate the mélange of grilled vegetable leftovers into your meals.

Sandwiches

FOR MANY PEOPLE sandwiches are a way of life—or at least a way of *lunch*. However, sandwiches work better in your diet if you eat them only occasionally. At those times, you can enjoy a variety. Here are some blood type–friendly combinations that you can try. They all contain Highly Beneficial or Neutral ingredients.

Place the sandwich fillings either on the commercially made Ezekiel or Essene breads, or on slices of those loaves you make yourself. The sandwiches based on vegetables and cheese are especially good on spelt baguettes. For roll-up sandwiches, or "wraps" as they're popularly called, you can make your own flour tortillas or crêpes. There is also a wide variety of pitas and flat breads available. Don't hesitate to serve these elegant and filling sandwiches to company or to your family when you're pressed for time. With a bowl of soup and a simple salad, these sandwiches can be a sumptuous treat for dinner.

Grilled Peppers (all varieties) and Goat Cheese	Blood Types O, B
Grilled Eggplant and Feta Cheese	Blood Types A, AB
Sliced Tomatoes, Fresh Mozzarella, and Basil	Blood Types O, AB
Braised Red Peppers and Onions with Feta	Blood Types O, B
Roasted Red Peppers and Goat Cheese	Blood Types O

Grilled Eggplant, Braised Shiitake Mushrooms, and Goat Cheese	Blood Type B
Almond Butter and Sliced Banana	Blood Types O, B
Peanut Butter, Raisins, and Honey	Blood Types A, AB
Tofu, Avocado, Alfalfa Sprouts, Lemon Vinaigrette	Blood Type A
Tofu, Tomato, Chopped Olives, Lemon Vinaigrette	Blood Type AB
Sunflower Butter and Plum Preserves	Blood Types O, A
Persimmons, Tahini, and Sprouts	Blood Types O, A
Grilled Chicken Breast	Blood Types O, A
Sliced Lamb with Mango or Peach Chutney	Blood Types O, B

These are acceptable for ALL blood types:

Fresh Mozzarella, Sautéed Zucchini, and Garlic

Ricotta, Chopped Walnuts, Raisins, and Honey

Soft Goat Cheese and Preserves

Mashed Sardines and Minced Garlic

Quick Tuna Salad (see page 283)

Curried Egg Salad (see page 283)

Turkey Burgers on Spelt Buns

Quick Common-Sense Suggestions

GRILLED OR ROASTED PEPPER
ON RYE CRACKERS WITH CHÈVRE

HIGHLY BENEFICIAL		NEUTRAL	O, B	AVOID	A, AB

2 red or yellow peppers, grilled or roasted with some olive oil
4 Rye Crisp crackers (TYPE O) *or rice crackers* (TYPE B)
2 oz. crumbled goat cheese

Slice peppers to size of cracker. Crumble goat cheese on top. *Serves 2.*

GRILLED GOAT CHEDDAR
ON EZEKIEL OR SPELT BREAD

HIGHLY BENEFICIAL	B, AB	NEUTRAL	O, A	AVOID	

2 slices Ezekiel bread
3 to 4 slices goat Cheddar
2 tablespoons butter or soft canola-oil margarine

Spread butter or margarine on one slice of bread, add goat cheese. Slice sandwich on the diagonal.   *Serves 1.*

CURRIED EGG SALAD

HIGHLY BENEFICIAL	O	NEUTRAL	A, B, AB	AVOID	

4 hard-boiled eggs, peeled and mashed
2 tablespoons Olive-Oil Mayonnaise (see page 318)

1 teaspoon salt or to taste
1 teaspoon good-quality curry powder

Mix all ingredients together and serve with Ezekiel bread or rice crackers.   *Serves 3.*

QUICK TUNA SALAD

HIGHLY BENEFICIAL	AB	NEUTRAL	O, A, B	AVOID	

1 can chunk light tuna, packed in water
1 can solid white tuna, packed in water
2 tablespoons Olive-Oil Mayonnaise (see page 318)
1 scallion, thinly sliced or ¼ red onion, diced

Drain tuna, but leave some liquid. Mix all ingredients well and serve on spelt toast. For a tuna melt, add any acceptable cheese. Soy cheese slices are also quite good.   *Serves 2.*

Eggs

EGGS HAVE RECEIVED a lot of bad press over the last few years. Many people have banished them from their diets. All of that cholesterol! Well, further research has proven that it's not the cholesterol in the egg; it's how the body produces cholesterol that accounts for harmful or healthy levels of dietary cholesterol in an individual. As a result of this new information, a lot of nutritionists are backpedaling, and eggs have been returned to the list of good foods we should eat, albeit on a limited basis.

Fried, poached, scrambled, soft-boiled, hard-boiled, or in omelettes and frittatas, eggs are little powerhouses of protein. Enjoy them according to the frequency recommended for your blood type and your particular health needs.

SINGLE-EGG OMELET

HIGHLY BENEFICIAL		NEUTRAL	O, A, B, AB	AVOID	

1 tablespoon olive oil
1 small green zucchini, washed and grated
1 large organic egg
2 fresh basil leaves
2 tablespoons grated romano
salt

In a medium frying pan, heat oil over medium heat and quickly cook zucchini 2 to 3 minutes, then set aside on a plate. Briskly beat egg, add 1 tablespoon water, and beat again. The idea is to get the egg as fluffy as possible. Add another bit of olive oil to grease the pan and reheat. Pour in egg, letting egg run around the whole bottom of the pan. Since there's only 1 egg, it's bound to be thin. Quickly add the zucchini, basil, and romano cheese. With a spatula, lift the edges of the omelet and carefully fold over the filling to make a half moon. Roll the omelet out of the pan and onto the plate. Season with salt to taste. *Serves 1.*

Alternative Fillings for
Omelets and Frittatas

With just a little forethought, any vegetables left over from yesterday's meal can become the filling for a breakfast or lunch egg dish.

If you've run out of ideas for fillings, remember that almost anything will do. Here's a short list of ideas that may inspire you!

Asparagus
Braised collards
Broccoli

Steamed carrots
Freshly grated carrot with crumbled goat cheese
  and fresh dill
Sautéed onions
Tomato and basil
Tofu, scallion, and cilantro
Wild rice tempeh with basmati rice

Be sure to warm any of your leftovers before using them to fill an omelet.

Tarts

TARTS ARE EASY to put together at the last moment once the tart shells have been made. And if you make the dough ahead and freeze it, you've provided yourself access to one of the quickest and easiest meals—or desserts—to prepare. Tarts can also make excellent hors d'oeuvres.

WHOLE-GRAIN DOUGH FOR CRUSTS AND SHELLS

HIGHLY BENEFICIAL		NEUTRAL	O, A, B, AB	AVOID	

1½ cups white spelt flour
½ cup whole-spelt flour
½ teaspoon salt
2 tablespoons sugar for a dessert crust (optional)
1 stick unsalted butter, cold, cut into small pieces, plus 3 tablespoons margarine (TYPES A AND AB SHOULD USE ALL MARGARINE)
4 to 5 tablespoons cold water

In a large mixing bowl, combine both flours and salt. If making a dessert tart, add the sugar. Cut in cold butter or margarine, working the flour into the butter using your fingertips. When mixture resembles coarse meal, begin to add water, 1 tablespoon at a time. It may not take all the water. The dough should be moist enough to form a ball, but not too wet. Wrap in plastic wrap and chill in the refrigerator for at least 2 hours. At this juncture, the dough will last for 5 days.

When ready to use dough, remove it from the refrigerator and let it sit for 45 minutes. Slice in two, and roll out on a floured board to ⅛-inch thickness. Cut dough into a circle and brush with olive oil. Pierce with a fork at intervals over the surface. Bake on a cookie sheet in a 350-degree oven for 5 to 8 minutes. Let cool.

Another option is to place cut-out circles of dough in 3- or 4-inch pie pans and form into shells. Dust the shell with flour and place a protective wrap over them. Repeat and stack, then either refrigerate or freeze. You can store the baked crust or raw pie shells in an airtight container in the refrigerator for a couple of days.

ARTICHOKE AND VIDALIA ONION TART

HIGHLY BENEFICIAL	O, A	NEUTRAL		AVOID	B, AB

1 baked tart shell
1 Vidalia onion, thinly sliced
1 tablespoon olive oil
2 cooked artichoke hearts, fresh or leftover, sliced
2 tablespoons crumbled goat cheese
salt and pepper

Sauté onion in the oil until lightly caramelized. Cool. Top tart shell with onion, sliced artichoke, and goat cheese. Add salt and pepper to taste. *Serves 2.*

EGGPLANT AND ROASTED-PEPPER TART

HIGHLY BENEFICIAL	B	NEUTRAL		AVOID	O, A, AB

1 baked tart shell
1 teaspoon Garlic-Shallot Mixture (see page 334)
or 1 clove garlic, peeled and pressed
1 small eggplant, grilled and sliced
1 roasted red pepper, sliced
1 tablespoon chopped fresh parsley
1 tablespoon olive oil

Distribute the Garlic-Shallot Mixture over the tart shell. Layer the tart with sliced eggplant and sliced pepper. Sprinkle with parsley, then drizzle with olive oil.   *Serves 2.*

PORTOBELLO MUSHROOM AND ONION TART

HIGHLY BENEFICIAL		NEUTRAL	O, A, B, AB	AVOID	

1 baked tart shell
2 tablespoons olive oil
1 onion, peeled and sliced
1 Portobello mushroom, stem removed and sliced
1 tablespoon chopped parsley
salt

Heat oil in a skillet over medium heat and gently cook onion until wilted. Add mushroom and cook another 5 to 8 minutes. Cool. Top tart shell with vegetables. Sprinkle with parsley and a pinch of salt.   *Serves 2.*

Frittatas

FRITTATAS ARE a very nice change from omelets. Though comprised of many of the same ingredients, frittatas are really quite different. They are generally more substantial, and their cooking methods can vary. Frittatas can be baked, cooked on top of the stove, and browned under the broiler. Whichever way frittatas are made, they all contain a singular element: satisfaction. They're fast, and pleasing to the eye. Most important, they appease the palate.

FRITTATA WITH PASTA AND CARAMELIZED ONION

HIGHLY BENEFICIAL		NEUTRAL	O, A, B, AB	AVOID	

This is a perfect way to use up any cooked spaghetti. It's also worth making just for this purpose.

¼ cup olive oil
1 fist-sized onion, finely chopped
2 to 3 cups cooked spaghetti (buckwheat, spelt, or rice)
4 eggs
salt
2 tablespoons butter, canola-oil margarine, or olive oil
handful chopped fresh parsley

Heat oil in a heavy, cast-iron skillet over low heat. Add onions, turning to coat with oil. Over low heat, cook onions until they become a beautiful golden brown. This will take quite some time, and they'll need to be stirred frequently. Transfer onions to a large bowl, add spaghetti, and mix well. In a small bowl, beat eggs until light, add a pinch of salt, then pour eggs over the spaghetti and onions. Mix them well. Wipe away any traces of onions or oil left in the skillet, turn heat to medium, and add butter or margarine. When hot, pour in egg mixture and spread it evenly over bottom of skillet. Cook about 5 minutes. Check bottom of frittata once or twice to be sure eggs are cooking thoroughly and frittata is turning a golden, crispy brown. When you are satisfied that the bottom is cooked through, you can either flip the frittata over, much as you would a pancake, or put it under the broiler for a moment, and cook until there is no more uncooked egg. Watch that it doesn't burn. Serve hot or let cook for a few minutes. Cut into wedges and sprinkle with parsley.   *Serves 4 to 6.*

ZUCCHINI & MUSHROOM FRITTATA

HIGHLY BENEFICIAL		NEUTRAL	O, A, B, AB	AVOID	

3 tablespoons olive oil
2 shallots or ½ small onion, chopped
2 medium zucchini, cut lengthwise, then
crosswise on the diagonal
1 Portobello mushroom, sliced
5 eggs
¼ cup grated romano cheese
salt

Preheat oven 350 degrees F. In a large heavy skillet, heat 1 tablespoon oil over medium heat and gently cook shallots. Add zucchini and sliced mushroom and cook until soft. Meanwhile beat eggs with a tablespoon of water. Add cheese and vegetables to the egg mixture. Mix well. Add remaining 2 tablespoons oil to skillet. When oil is hot, add egg mixture. Cook on low heat until half done, then finish cooking in the oven. The frittata will puff up nicely. Salt to taste.   *Serves 4 to 6.*

SPINACH FRITTATA

HIGHLY BENEFICIAL	O, A	NEUTRAL	B, AB	AVOID	

For a decidedly Greek flavor in this delicious frittata, use some good-quality feta cheese. Or use ¼ cup grated romano.

5 eggs
1 tablespoon water
1 bunch spinach, washed, dried and finely chopped
2 tablespoons olive oil
1 tablespoon Garlic-Shallot Mixture (see page 334)
¼ cup crumbled feta or grated romano cheese
squeeze of lemon juice (optional)
salt

Preheat broiler. Beat eggs with water. Add the spinach. In a large skillet, heat oil over medium heat and cook shallot mixture until softened. Add spinach-egg mixture all at once and cook over medium heat until almost done. While the top is still a bit runny, top with cheese and run under the broiler until done, about 2 or 3 minutes. Season with a squeeze of lemon, salt, and serve.   *Serves 4 to 6.*

Crêpes, or French Pancakes

THIS RECIPE IS an adaptation of an old French standby. It uses white spelt flour instead of wheat flour, and soy milk rather than dairy milk, but the results are satisfyingly similar. Crêpes are very versatile. They can be eaten as is with fruit jam or a dusting of sugar. They can be filled and rolled with braised vegetables, poultry, tofu, or almost anything else you can imagine. The world of crêpes is hardly confined to the French. Russian crêpes are called *blinis*, Jewish crêpes are called *blintzes*. They can also be prepared well ahead of time, and then reheated with other leftovers. This recipe is good for all blood types. What you decide to eat with your crêpes should be as well.

CRÊPES

HIGHLY BENEFICIAL		NEUTRAL	O, A, B, AB	AVOID	

2 eggs
1 cup soy milk (TYPE B SHOULD SUBSTITUTE DAIRY)
½ teaspoon salt
2 tablespoons melted butter, cooled, or margarine
1 cup white spelt flour
1 to 2 tablespoons water to thin batter (if necessary)
light olive oil or canola oil for pan

In a mixing bowl, beat eggs well. Add soy milk, salt, melted butter or margarine, and flour; mix well. Let sit 20 minutes. If you don't have a crêpe pan, and few people do, use an 8- or 9-inch skillet. Heat skillet until moderately hot, then grease with a minimum of oil, using a paper towel to wipe up excess. With a ladle or large serving spoon, pour batter into skillet. Quickly tilt pan in a circular motion to evenly and thinly spread batter. Cook for a few minutes, until the edges of crêpe pull away from sides. Then, with a long spatula, lift one side and carefully flip crêpe over. Cook for one more minute, then flip onto a plate. Repeat process, using the oiled paper towel to grease the pan for each new crêpe. Fill with fresh fruit or jam, cooked vegetables from last night's dinner, or sautéed berries, or use to make wraps. *Yields about 8 pancakes.*

SEVENTEEN

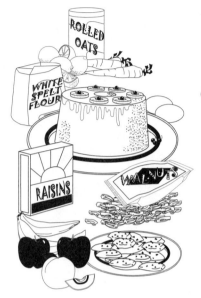

Desserts, Cheese, & Fruit

*D*ESSERTS ARE OFTEN AT THE CENTER OF CHILD-hood memories, family celebrations, and holidays. Cakes, cookies, pies, tarts, and ice creams are *de rigueur* for many people. It is a universal truth that many people refuse to go a day without a sweet of some kind. But cakes and cookies aren't the only things people love to eat for dessert. Combinations of fruits and cheeses make light desserts. A ripe Anjou pear, a rich baked apple, a runny cheese—these are simple and satisfying conclusions.

Encourage children to view dessert as a real treat, and be sure to make it one. Purchase only the best ice creams, preferably organic. Make your own cookies, cakes, and pies. In this way, you are able to control the ingredients. Most families have favorite desserts. If yours doesn't yet, then establish a traditional family favorite.

Try to avoid buying commercially made baked goods. Read the nutrition label and list of ingredients. You'll see that all commercial goods are made with wheat flour, many are made with tropical oils, and most contain chemical ingredients that the majority of people can't even pronounce. That will usually stop most health-minded people right there. At least it should!

A homemade dessert can be a terrific treat. The only real problem is overindulgence. If three or four dozen cookies are lurking in the kitchen, many people feel a responsibility to eat them before they get stale or go bad. Freezing extra cookies sometimes helps, although frozen cookies don't take very long to defrost. In the world of desserts, the best advice is a gentle word or two: *A little goes a long way.*

WALNUT COOKIES

HIGHLY BENEFICIAL		NEUTRAL	O, B	AVOID	A, AB

These rich, not too sweet cookies are delicious served with a piece of ripe fruit. They make a wonderful light dessert. There are only five ingredients, so they're easy to put together.

1 stick butter
¼ cup sugar
1 cup walnuts, finely chopped
1 cup spelt flour
confectioners' sugar

Preheat oven to 350 degrees F. Butter cookie sheets. In a mixing bowl, cream butter and sugar. Add nuts and flour and stir to combine. Drop by teaspoonfuls about 2 inches apart onto prepared cookie sheets. Bake approximately 25 minutes. Keep a careful watch after the first 20 minutes to make sure that the

cookies don't get darker than golden. You want them to be golden brown. With spatula immediately remove from pans and cool on wire rack. Sprinkle lightly with sugar.
Makes 20 to 30 cookies.

CARROT-GINGER RAISIN CAKE

HIGHLY BENEFICIAL		NEUTRAL	O, A, AB	AVOID	B

This spicy cake has both a great taste and texture. It is ideal for a birthday cake, especially with the Goat-Cheese Frosting.

butter, margarine, or oil for pans
2 cups whole-spelt flour
2 teaspoons baking soda
2 teaspoons baking powder
1 teaspoon salt
1⅓ cup canola oil
1½ cups light brown sugar
4 eggs, slightly beaten
3 cups grated carrots
2-inch piece fresh ginger, peeled and grated
½ cup raisins
1 cup chopped walnuts

Preheat oven to 325 degrees F. Grease and flour two 8-inch round cake pans. In a large mixing bowl, mix dry ingredients together. In another bowl, combine oil, sugar, eggs, carrots, and ginger. Add carrot mixture to dry ingredients and with a minimum of folding, combine them. Stir in raisins and walnuts. *Do not overmix.* Fill prepared pans almost to the top. Bake 55 minutes, or until a cake tester comes out clean. Let cool and remove cakes from pan. This cake can be served plain, dusted with confectioners' sugar, or frosted with Goat-Cheese Frosting.   *Makes two 8-inch rounds.*

GOAT-CHEESE FROSTING

HIGHLY BENEFICIAL		NEUTRAL	O, A, B, AB	AVOID	

4 oz. goat cheese, softened to room temperature
2 oz. butter or canola-oil margarine, softened to room
temperature
¾ cup confectioners' sugar
2 tablespoons honey
1 tablespoon rice milk
1 teaspoon vanilla extract (TYPES A, B, AB)
or almond extract (TYPE O)
½ teaspoon lemon zest

In a small bowl, blend goat cheese and butter using a fork. Add confectioners' sugar and blend in, but don't whip. Fold in honey, rice milk, vanilla or almond extract, and lemon zest. Spread on cooled cake. Refrigerate if not served immediately. *Makes about 1½ cups.*

WALNUT SHORTBREAD

HIGHLY BENEFICIAL		NEUTRAL	O, B	AVOID	A, AB

This is another simple but rich dessert that complements fruit salad, poached fruit, or a bunch of grapes.

1 cup butter, at room temperature
1½ cups spelt flour (TYPE B CAN SUBSTITUTE
½ CUP OAT FLOUR FOR ½ CUP SPELT)
½ cup walnuts, ground in blender
½ cup confectioners' sugar
pinch of salt

Preheat oven to 350 degrees F. In large mixing bowl, cream butter. Add flour, walnuts, sugar, and salt and stir until blended. The dough will be very stiff. Press dough firmly with your fingers into ungreased 9 x 9 inch-pan. Prick entire surface at ½-inch intervals with a fork to let out steam. Bake 25 minutes, or until just golden. Remove from oven, allow to cool a few minutes, then cut into squares or narrow rectangles. If you make this in a pie dish of approximately the same square-inch measurement, cut into triangles.   *Makes 12 to 16 pieces.*

CYBER RECIPE

TOFU CHOCOLATE MOUSSE

AUTHOR: Holly Allen (Holly3325@juno.com)

TYPE A

A great dessert for chocoholics. But, if restricted, it's great without chocolate, and can be flavored with various extracts, used as a garnish for fresh fruit, or sprinkled on top of allowed cereals (granola).

1 (10-oz.) pkg. firm, silken tofu, drained
¼ cup light honey
¼ cup fruit syrup
½ teaspoon ground cinnamon
1 teaspoon instant coffee
2 tablespoons cocoa
½ teaspoon vanilla

Purée all the ingredients until thoroughly mixed. Place in a refrig-type bowl with a tight cover. Cover and chill 4 to 5 hours. Enjoy!   *Serves 2.*

LEMON SQUARES

HIGHLY BENEFICIAL		NEUTRAL	O, B	AVOID	A, AB

Lemon squares are both tart and sweet—and rich. Cut the squares into fairly small pieces.

¾ cup spelt flour
¼ cup walnuts, ground in blender
¼ cup confectioners' sugar
½ cup melted butter, cooled
¾ cup granulated sugar
½ teaspoon baking powder
2 eggs, beaten
3 tablespoons lemon juice
3 teaspoons grated lemon peel
pinch of salt

Preheat oven to 350 degrees F. In a small bowl, stir flour, walnuts, and confectioners' sugar until blended. Add butter and combine well. Press dough firmly with your fingers into 8 x 8-inch buttered pan. Bake until lightly colored, about 20 minutes.

While pastry is baking, combine granulated sugar, baking powder, eggs, lemon juice, lemon peel, and salt in a mixing bowl. Beat well for just a moment. Pour over warm, not hot, pastry and return to oven for another 20 minutes, or until lemon topping is slightly puffed, firm, and a lovely gold. Cut into 2-inch squares when cool. *Makes 12 to 16 pieces.*

SPELT BREAD PUDDING

HIGHLY BENEFICIAL		NEUTRAL	A, B, AB	AVOID	O

Spelt bread pudding began as an inedible loaf of whole-spelt French bread. As was mentioned in the "Breads" section, many attempts have to be made in the bread-baking process before a good loaf of bread is achieved. What to do with hard and heavy loaves? Milk and eggs solved the problem. Stale bread can be used for puddings, bread crumbs, croutons, and *chapons*, which are small rectangular pieces of stale bread, rubbed with garlic, that accompany mesclun and Niçoise salads. Hearty slices of stale bread also make good thickeners for soups. Place a slice or two at the bottom of the bowl, ladle in some soup, and let soak. Also, this pudding doubles as an excellent quick breakfast.

> *about 5 cups stale spelt bread cubes*
> *5 cups milk or soy milk*
> *butter for pan*
> *4 eggs or egg substitute*
> *1½ cups sugar*
> *3 tablespoons vanilla extract*
> *juice and grated rind of 1 lemon*
> *pinch of salt*
> *1 cup dried cherries*

Place bread in bowl, cover with milk, and let sit 45 minutes. Preheat oven to 325 degrees F. Butter a 9 x 13 x 2-inch glass baking pan. Beat eggs until light. Add sugar, vanilla, lemon juice, lemon rind, and salt, and beat well. Pour into bread and milk mixture. Stir in cherries. Pour into prepared pan and bake 1 hour, or until set. Can be eaten warm or cold.   *Serves 12.*

🍴 CYBER RECIPE 🍴

CUSTARD PIE (DAIRYLESS)
AUTHOR: Karen Watland (kswatland@aol.com)

TYPE A

If you love custard you will love this one!

5 eggs
3 cups soy milk
⅓ cup sugar (you may try other sweetener substitutes)
1 tablespoon vanilla
½ teaspoon nutmeg
prebaked pie crust

Preheat oven to 450 degrees F. Beat eggs slightly. Scald soy milk (important). Beat soy milk, sugar, vanilla, and nutmeg into eggs. Pour into pie shell. Sprinkle a little nutmeg on top for color. Pour remaining custard into dishes and place in pan of water set on lower rack of oven. Bake filled pie crust on upper rack of oven 15 minutes, then reduce temperature to 350 degrees and bake another 10 minutes. To test pie for doneness use a table knife inserted into pie. If knife comes out clean it is done. Set a clean dish towel on pie after you bring it out of oven and place it on a cooling rack. *Serves 8.*

CRANBERRY BISCOTTI

HIGHLY BENEFICIAL		NEUTRAL	O, A, B, AB	AVOID	

Cranberry *biscotti* make a wonderful tasty Christmas cookie as well as a good teething biscuit for babies.

Dip the biscotti in your tea or coffee. Cranberries add a chewy, tart sweetness.

> *butter or oil for cookie sheet*
> *3 eggs*
> *¼ cup sugar*
> *3 tablespoons butter or margarine, melted and cooled*
> *1 teaspoon vanilla* (Types A, B, and AB)
> *1 teaspoon almond extract* (Type O)
> *zest of 1 lemon or orange*
> *1 tablespoon pineapple juice*
> *1⅔ cups spelt flour*
> *1 teaspoon baking powder*
> *¼ teaspoon salt*
> *¼ teaspoon nutmeg* (Type O omit)
> *½ cup chopped fresh cranberries*
> *egg wash for glaze (made from 1 beaten egg)*

Preheat oven to 350 degrees F. Grease cookie sheet. Beat eggs until foamy, then slowly add sugar, beating until light. Add shortening, vanilla, lemon zest, and pineapple juice. In a separate bowl, mix all dry ingredients. Add dry ingredients to egg mixture and blend well. Stir in cranberries. The dough will be soft. Divide dough in half. On a prepared cookie sheet, mold each half into a long thin loaf, about 8 by 3 inches. Bake 25 minutes. Remove from oven and reduce heat to 325 degrees F. Let loaves cool 10 minutes. Place loaves on a cutting board and slice on the diagonal, into 1½-inch-thick pieces. Return cookies to cookie sheet and toast on one side, 5 minutes, then turn each cookie and toast on the other side another 10 minutes. Remove from oven when golden brown. Store for a week in a cookie jar.   *Makes 32 pieces.*

RICE-CRISPY CAKES

HIGHLY BENEFICIAL		NEUTRAL	O, A, B, AB	AVOID	

This crispy, chewy rice treat is an all-time favorite of children everywhere. Crispy cakes are palate pleasers, and these are every bit as sweet and delectable as the commercial versions.

2 tablespoons butter or canola-oil margarine
(depending on Type)
¼ cup honey, maple syrup, or brown rice syrup
2 tablespoons brown sugar
¼ tablespoon salt
3 cups crispy rice cereal (brown rice is the nuttiest)

In a 3-quart saucepan, melt butter or margarine, honey or other liquid sweetener, sugar, and salt. Add rice cereal all at once and stir to incorporate thoroughly. Immediately press mixture into a flat, rectangular plastic or glass container. A 5 x 8-inch dish works well. The cakes should be about 1 inch high by 2 inches square. Unlike those made with marshmallows, these must be refrigerated to hold together.   *Makes 16 bars.*

PEANUT BUTTER COOKIES

HIGHLY BENEFICIAL		NEUTRAL	A, AB	AVOID	O, B

The fact that peanuts are listed as Highly Beneficial is always a good reason to mix up a batch of these rich and flavorful cookies. They're not too sweet, so if you'd like them sweeter, add an extra ¼ cup sugar.

grease or parchment paper for cookie sheets
½ cup margarine
½ cup brown sugar
¼ cup white sugar
2 eggs
1¼ cups chunky, unsalted peanut butter
generous pinch of salt
½ teaspoon baking soda
1 teaspoon vanilla extract
1 cup spelt flour
½ cup oat flour

Preheat oven to 350 degrees F. Grease cookie sheets. Beat margarine until soft, then add sugars and beat until creamy. Beat in eggs, peanut butter, salt, baking soda, and vanilla, fully incorporating all the peanut butter. Stir in both flours, mixing well. Roll dough between your palms into 1-inch balls and place on greased cookie sheet, or unbuttered parchment paper. Flatten to about ¼-inch with the tines of a fork. Bake 7 to 10 minutes, or until cookies begin to color. Cool on wire racks. *Makes about 40 cookies.*

APPLE CAKE

HIGHLY BENEFICIAL		NEUTRAL	O, A, B, AB	AVOID	

This is a rich but not overly sweet cake. If you'd prefer a slightly sweeter cake, add a little more sugar. Type A and Type AB can substitute canola-oil margarine.

2 to 2½ cups peeled and thinly sliced apples
¾ cup sugar
juice and grated rind of 1 lemon
1 tablespoon spelt flour
5 tablespoons melted butter or margarine
½ cup white spelt flour
½ cup whole-spelt flour
1 teaspoon baking powder
pinch of salt
2 eggs or egg substitute
¼ cup soy milk

Preheat oven to 350 degrees F. Butter bottom of an 8- or 9-inch pie pan deep enough to hold all the batter. Arrange apple slices in an attractive pattern in the pie pan. When cake has finished cooking, it will be inverted on a plate. Sprinkle apples with ½ cup sugar, lemon juice, and grated lemon rind. Type A and Type AB can sprinkle the fruit with cinnamon. Type B can sprinkle nutmeg. Dust with a tablespoon of flour, then pour melted butter or margarine over apples.

In a bowl, combine both flours, remaining ¼ cup sugar, baking powder, and salt. In another bowl, beat eggs until light, then quickly stir in remaining tablespoon melted butter and soy milk. Add liquid ingredients to flour mixture and blend with as few strokes as possible. Pour batter over apples into pie pan. Bake 30 to 40 minutes, until golden brown and a straw comes out clean. Cover with a serving platter and reverse. *Serves 8 to 10.*

BASMATI RICE PUDDING

HIGHLY BENEFICIAL		NEUTRAL	O, A, B, AB	AVOID	

This rice pudding is a pleasant alternative to the usual milk-based ones. It's a good way to use up any leftover rice in your refrigerator. Try this substantial pudding for lunch with a fruit salad. It's also a healthy cold breakfast pudding. Quick, too!

butter for baking dish
2 cups basmati rice, cooked
4 eggs
2 cups soy milk
½ cup sugar
2 tablespoons melted butter or canola-oil margarine
grated rind of 1 lemon
juice of ½ lemon
½ cup raisins

Preheat oven to 350 degrees F. Grease baking dish and add rice. In large mixing bowl, beat eggs with a whisk until frothy. Add remaining ingredients and mix thoroughly. Pour mixture over rice, combining well with a fork. Bake pudding until set, approximately 40 to 50 minutes.   *Serves 6 to 8.*

PINEAPPLE UPSIDE-DOWN CAKE

HIGHLY BENEFICIAL		NEUTRAL	O, A, B, AB	AVOID	

This is an old favorite. You'll swear that this version is just like the kind mother used to make.

¼ cup butter or canola-oil margarine
½ cup brown sugar
6 to 9 slices canned, drained unsweetened pineapple
enough small pieces of fruit to fit into the pineapple "holes";
try halved pitted cherries or halved pitted apricots
1 cup white spelt flour
1 teaspoon baking powder
4 eggs
2 tablespoons melted butter or margarine
¾ cup sugar

Preheat oven to 350 degrees F. In a 9-inch round, cast-iron skillet, melt butter or margarine. Add sugar, stirring well. Distribute this mixture evenly over bottom of skillet. Turn off heat and add pineapple slices, fitting them neatly around perimeter of skillet, and placing 1 slice in middle. Fill the "holes" with fruit of your choice. In a medium bowl, mix spelt flour and baking powder well. In a smaller bowl, beat eggs until light. Add melted butter or margarine, then sugar, and beat until well blended. Add liquid to dry ingredients and stir until well blended. Pour batter over pineapple. Bake approximately 25 to 30 minutes, until cake is golden. Remove cake from oven. Place a large plate over skillet, and turn cake upside down. Leave on counter a few minutes, with skillet still upside down over plate, to let cake settle. Carefully remove skillet to reveal pineapple and fruit topping. *Serves 6 to 9.*

🍴 C Y B E R   R E C I P E 🍴

CAROB ALMOND COOKIES
AUTHOR: Judy R. (rudin003@gold.tc.umn.edu)

ALL BLOOD TYPES

This recipe is the result of my attempts to develop a decent cookie that would be appropriate for Type Os and would also be suitable for yeast- and sugar-free diets. These cookies are slightly sweet, very carob-y, and have a really nice cakelike texture. They're fine as a dessert, but given their ingredients, you could also eat them as part of a healthy breakfast!

⅓ cup almond butter
2 tablespoons oil
1½ large apples (pears can also be used)
2 eggs
¼ teaspoon unbuttered, corn-free vitamin C crystals
1¼ cups brown rice flour or 1 cup brown rice flour
plus ¼ cup spelt or kamut flour
¾ teaspoon baking soda
(1 teaspoon of your favorite baking powder can be
substituted for the vitamin C and baking soda)
¾ cup carob powder
¼ teaspoon salt
about 30 whole almonds (optional)

Oil 2 cookie sheets and preheat oven to 350 degrees F. Chop apples into small chunks and put in blender. Add almond butter, oil, eggs, and vitamin C crystals. Purée everything together. You may need to push the apples down a few times to get them started. If more liquid is needed to make the purée, add a bit of water. In a separate bowl, combine flour, baking soda (or baking powder, if you are not using the vitamin C crystals and baking soda), carob powder and salt; mix well. Add the purée to the dry ingredients and stir just until everything is well blended. Drop by rounded tablespoonsful onto the cookie sheets. Bake 10 to 12 minutes. Cookies are done when a toothpick inserted in the center comes out dry. Allow to cool for 5 minutes. *Makes 24 cookies.*

TOFU-BANANA PUDDING

HIGHLY BENEFICIAL		NEUTRAL	O	AVOID	A, B, AB

This fat-free pudding is easy to make and is a satisfying light dessert. Children love it, too. Try it for breakfast!

1 cake tofu
2 ripe bananas

Combine ingredients in a blender and purée a few moments. Pour into individual little bowls and chill. *Serves 2 to 4.*

TOFU-PUMPKIN PUDDING

HIGHLY BENEFICIAL	O, A, AB	NEUTRAL		AVOID	B

The variations for this simple tofu treat are endless. It's a terrific way to get your soy and some healthy fruit all at the same time. So smooth and satisfying, too.

1 cake tofu
1 cup canned pumpkin
honey as needed (start with 1 to 2 tablespoons)

Purée all of the ingredients in a blender, pour into bowls, and chill.   *Serves 3 to 4.*

Cheese

CHEESE HAS long been a classic way to end a lovely meal, and there are countless cheeses available today. However, cow's milk causes a lot of problems for certain blood types, chief among them the increased production of mucus. Type O and Type A do best to eliminate dairy almost completely from their diets, with a few exceptions given for sheep and goat cheese. Type B and Type AB are allowed a much wider variety of cow's milk cheeses. If you don't have a selection of sheep and goat cheese in your local market, ask for it. Offer to buy it in bulk, and recruit friends to share the purchase with you. Cheese is high in saturated fat, so go easy. Type B is the only blood type for whom cheese is really beneficial. When you purchase cheese, be sure to read the label. For example, not all feta cheese is made from goat's milk. Sometimes cow's milk is used.

Here is a list of the many goat and sheep cheeses. Check your blood type chart before eating.

Goat's Milk Cheeses
Crottin
Hollandse chèvre
Montrâchet
Chèvrotin
Chavrie
Feta
Boucheron
Pyramide

Coach Farms
Ile de France

Sheep's Milk Cheeses
Roquefort
Feta
Pecorino romano
Saint Thèrese
Brigantine
Manchego
Ricotta salata
Tomes

Fruit

FRUIT IS AMONG nature's sweetest gifts. The quality and flavor of fruit in season can be spectacular. Fruit makes a lovely companion to cheese for a classic dessert. It is the perfect snack between meals, an ideal addition to any meal, and can indeed be eaten as a meal. If children are hungry late in the afternoon, give them a piece of fruit an hour before their supper.

SAUTÉED PEARS OR APPLES

HIGHLY BENEFICIAL		NEUTRAL	O, A, B, AB	AVOID	

Sautéeing ripe pears and apples is a good way to use fruit that you might otherwise not eat out of hand. This is a simple fall dessert or a sublime topping for crêpes or pancakes. It is also wonderful served with cottage or ricotta cheese. Allow at least one pear or apple per person. A pinch of curry powder cooked in the butter or margarine adds a piquant flavor.

2 pears or apples
2 tablespoons butter (TYPE A AND TYPE AB CAN
USE SOY OR CANOLA-OIL MARGARINE)
cinnamon or nutmeg

Peel and thinly slice pears or apples. Melt butter in a heavy skillet over low heat. Add fruit, turning gently to coat with butter
or margarine. Turn heat very low and cover pan, stewing fruit
in butter or margarine and whatever juice the fruit throws off.
If there doesn't seem to be enough liquid, add a tablespoon of
water at a time. Cook 7 to 10 minutes, or until fruit is soft.
There should be a little syrup. Type A and Type AB can sprinkle with cinnamon or nutmeg. Type B can sprinkle the fruit
with nutmeg.   *Serves 2.*

SAUTÉED BANANAS

HIGHLY BENEFICIAL	B	NEUTRAL	0	AVOID	A, AB

Ripe bananas aren't appealing to some people. Rather than tossing them out, try turning them in a little butter. Surprising and
wonderful with curried dishes, they're also good for breakfast
with a little ricotta or fresh goat cheese. Serve with organic
vanilla ice cream. A triumph of tastes and textures, cold and hot.
Allow one banana per person.

2 ripe bananas
2 tablespoons butter
1 tablespoon lemon juice (optional)
grated lemon rind

Cut bananas in half crosswise, then cut in half lengthwise. The
bananas should be quartered. Melt butter in a heavy skillet.
Reduce heat to low and add bananas, turning carefully in the
butter. They will brown and get softer. Don't let them burn.

Cook 4 to 6 minutes. Sprinkle with lemon juice, if using, and lemon rind. Serve at once.   *Serves 2.*

FRESH FIG SALAD

HIGHLY BENEFICIAL	O, A, AB	NEUTRAL	B	AVOID	

Fresh figs are in season for a very short time. The Black Mission and Calmyrna figs are the most widely available, but there are over 150 varieties. Eat ripe figs out of hand, or serve them as presented here, with a creamy fresh goat cheese. Allow three to four figs and a slice or two of cheese per serving.

3 to 4 figs per person
goat cheese

Slice figs lengthwise, exposing the complex and lovely flesh. Fan the figs out on a plate, and top with bits of broken crumbled goat cheese.

TROPICAL SALAD

HIGHLY BENEFICIAL	O, A, B, AB	NEUTRAL		AVOID	

Combine these succulent and fragrant fruits according to your taste and blood type. A generous squeeze of lemon or lime juice will keep the colors intact, and the intense tartness is dressing enough for many people. If you prefer, swirl Ricotta Dressing (page 319) over the top of each portion for a richer version.

papaya (TYPES O, A, B, AND AB)
mango (TYPES O, B)
kiwi (TYPES O, A, B, AND AB)

pineapple (Types O, A, B, and AB)
carambola (star fruit) (Types O, A)
banana (Types O, B)
guava (Types O, A, B)
lemon or lime juice

Prepare all the fruit: Peel, seed, and cut the papaya and mango. Peel the kiwi and cut into slices or wedges. Cut pineapple into small chunks. Slice carambola so that each piece is a little star. Slice banana. Peel and slice guava. This salad can be layered in a glass bowl, each individual fruit in a single layer, or it can be very gently turned to mix the fruits. Sprinkle each layer with lemon or lime juice, or pour juice over salad before turning. *Allow about 1 cup prepared fruit per person.*

FRUIT COMPOTE

HIGHLY BENEFICIAL	O, A, B, AB NEUTRAL	AVOID

Poaching fruit is an excellent way to use very ripe fruit. Don't be afraid to use some dried prunes and apricots to the mix, either. Combinations are endless, so be creative! Poached fruit over yogurt or ricotta makes a lovely breakfast or a light lunch.

1 cup water
¾ cup sugar
juice and grated rind of 1 lemon
3 cloves
1 cup apples, pears, peaches, or plums
1 cup apricots, grapes, nectarines, or cherries
½ cup torn fresh mint leaves (optional)

A poaching syrup should be prepared first. In a large nonreactive saucepan, bring water to a boil, add sugar, lemon juice, lemon rind, and cloves. You don't have to peel the fruit if you don't want to. Remove all seeds and pits, slice larger fruit, and halve smaller ones, like apricots and plums. If you have a cherry pitter, leave cherries whole; if not, halve them as you remove the pits. Leave grapes whole. Add any combination of fruits to the boiling syrup, allowing 1 large and several smaller fruits per person. Poached, uncovered, about 10 to 15 minutes. Lift fruit carefully from syrup with a slotted spoon and place in a serving bowl. Continue to cook and reduce syrup another 8 to 10 minutes. Remove cloves and pour thickened syrup over fruits. Cool in refrigerator. Sprinkle with mint leaves, if desired. *Serves 2*.

BAKED APPLES

HIGHLY BENEFICIAL	O, A, AB	NEUTRAL	B	AVOID	

The best commercial apple for baking is the Rome. They are large, dry, and sweet, perfect for stuffing with a combination of nuts, dried fruits, and maple syrup. Just because other apples may not hold their shape so well as Romes, don't discriminate. Granny Smiths, Cortlands, and Fujis—all are delicious. Allow one apple per serving. Baked apples are great for breakfast, so cook extra. The proportions of nuts and fruits are general. Adjust according to taste.

4 apples
½ cup chopped walnuts
½ cup mixed dried figs and apricots
juice of ½ lemon
grated rind of ½ lemon
maple syrup
2 tablespoons butter or margarine
1 cup boiling water

Preheat oven to 350 degrees F. Core apples, taking care not to pierce the bottoms. Mix walnuts, dried fruit, lemon juice, and rind. Poor enough maple syrup over fruit-nut mixture to moisten well, about 2 tablespoons. Fill apples, without packing filling into too tightly. If filling mounds at the top of the apple, that's fine. Place a generous pat of butter or margarine on top of the filling and place apples in a glass baking dish. Pour boiling water into the dish around the apples. Bake 20 to 30 minutes, or until apples are tender. While they are baking, you can baste the apples with the pan juices. When apples are done, transfer them to a serving dish, pour liquid in pan into a small skillet, and reduce over medium-high heat until thickened. Spoon sauce over apples before serving.

One apple per serving.

APPLE PIE

HIGHLY BENEFICIAL		NEUTRAL	O, A, B, AB	AVOID	

This pie can be adapted to all blood types. Although apple is of Neutral value, it is a traditional American dessert, especially during the fall and the holidays.

PIE CRUST

1½ cup white spelt flour
½ cup whole-spelt flour
½ teaspoon salt
2 tablespoons sugar
1 stick unsalted butter, cubed (TYPE A AND TYPE AB
SHOULD USE ALL SOY OR CANOLA-OIL MARGARINE)
3 tablespoons margarine, cubed
5 tablespoons chilled water

FILLING

8 medium apples, Granny Smith or Ida Reds, if available
⅓ cup sugar
3 tablespoons spelt flour
⅛ teaspoon freshly grated nutmeg (TYPE O AVOID)
1 tablespoon lime juice
zest of 1 lime
2 tablespoons butter, cubed, for dotting (TYPE A AND TYPE AB
SHOULD USE SOY OR CANOLA-OIL MARGARINE)
1 egg, beaten, for glaze
sugar for sprinkling

Prepare pie crust: In a mixing bowl, combine flours, salt, and sugar. Cut in butter or margarine using your fingertips and blending well. The dough should resemble a coarse meal. Add water a little at a time, gently stirring with fork, until mixture forms a ball. Cover with plastic wrap and refrigerate at least 30 minutes. The dough will hold in the refrigerator for a couple of days, so if you are anticipating a holiday event, making the crust prepares you ahead of time.

Prepare filling: Peel and core apples; slice thinly. Add sugar, flour, and nutmeg, mixing well. Add lime juice and zest and mix well again. The filling may seem dry, but apples have a lot of moisture, and as they cook their juices will be released. The flour will thicken the juice, making a perfect pie filling.

Assemble the pie: Preheat oven to 350 degrees F. When ready to make pie, remove dough from refrigerator and let it sit at room temperature until soft enough to roll out, about 30 minutes. Cut dough into 2 pieces. Roll out 1 piece on a lightly floured surface, keeping the rolling pin dusted with spelt flour. Roll dough into a 12-inch circle, trimming if necessary. Roll half onto pin, lift up, and carefully roll out onto pie pan. Make sure the flattened dough is pressed down into bottom of pan, where it meets sides. Pierce crust with a fork, poking crust in many different places. Allow edges of dough to hang over sides of pan. Excess dough can be trimmed and crimped later.

Fill pie with apple mixture and dot with butter or margarine. Roll out remaining half of dough and gently place over the apples. Crimp crust by pinching both top and bottom pieces together. Trim off any excess. A little bit of water on the fingertips is a good binding agent. Brush with a beaten egg and sprinkle a little sugar over top. Cut a few air vents in top crust in any design you prefer. Bake on center rack of oven until crust is golden and juices are bubbling, at least 1 hour.   *Serves 8.*

EIGHTEEN

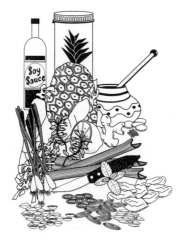

Dressings, Sauces, Chutneys, & Relishes

RESSING SEEMS AN IDEAL NAME FOR ALL THOSE side dishes that really do dress up other foods. We generally think of this rather extensive group as table condiments, but anyone who has ever had the taste of a dish brought alive with the introduction of a sauce or relish knows otherwise. These recipes will enable you to take something quick and easy, such as baked chicken, and transform it into something far more enticing, perhaps a Chicken with Mango-Ginger Chutney. A simple salad dressing can add a pleasant change and a nutritional boost to a fruit or mixed greens salad. Most of these recipes can be prepared very quickly. If you make them in advance and in quantity, it will be all the easier to serve a nutritious meal, even when you're pressed for time.

OLIVE-OIL MAYONNAISE

HIGHLY BENEFICIAL		NEUTRAL	O, A, B, AB	AVOID	

This is a basic mayonnaise that uses olive or canola oil and lemon or lime juice instead of vinegar. It is best to use a lighter olive oil as opposed to an extra-virgin. In this way, you achieve a flavor similar to that of canola. This mayonnaise should be used in all recipes calling for mayonnaise. CAUTION: Although many mayonnaise recipes call for the use of raw egg yolk, we suggest instead starting the recipe with a tablespoon or two of the canola-oil mayonnaise that can be found in most health-food markets. Since lemon juice is acidic, the theory of adding raw egg is that the juice cooks the egg, just as lemon or lime is used to cook the raw fish in seviche. However, the USDA no longer allows restaurants to use this method for two reasons: First, a lack of control in preparation, and second, the very real potential for food poisoning. Avoid eating raw egg at any of your meals.

1 or 2 tablespoons canola-oil mayonnaise
¼ teaspoon salt
2 tablespoons lime or lemon juice
1 cup light olive or canola oil

In a blender or food processor, make a basic mayonnaise by whipping the canola-oil mayonnaise and lemon juice together, and drizzling in the oil until it thickens. Keep chilled
Makes about 1½ cups.

RICOTTA DRESSING

HIGHLY BENEFICIAL	B, AB	NEUTRAL	A	AVOID	O

Thinned ricotta makes a creamy dressing for those fruit salads that are served as a complete meal rather than as a dessert.

1 cup ricotta cheese
2 tablespoons honey
1 tablespoon lemon juice
2 tablespoons pineapple juice (optional), for further thinning
grated rind of ½ lemon

In a small bowl, combine all ingredients and stir until thoroughly mixed.   *Makes 1½ cups.*

ALMOND DRESSING

HIGHLY BENEFICIAL		NEUTRAL	O, A, B, AB	AVOID	

Like tahini, almond butter can be thinned to make a delicious dressing for fruit salads.

½ cup almond butter
1 tablespoon honey
¼ cup water

In a small bowl, combine all ingredients and mix until well blended. Drizzle over fruit. Use more water if you want a thinner, lighter dressing.   *Makes ¾ cup.*

🍴 CYBER RECIPE 🍴

SOY CHEESE SAUCE

AUTHOR: Wayne Sander (wbsander@aol.com)

TYPES O, A, AB

Quick and easy cheese sauce for pasta or vegetables.

3 oz. Cheddar soy cheese
3 oz. silken tofu
2 tablespoons vegetable oil (linseed, canola, olive)
1 tablespoon soy milk or water
salt

Grate soy cheese and combine with remaining ingredients in a microwave-safe bowl. Blend well with an electric mixer. Microwave 30 seconds. Blend again and microwave another 30 seconds. As everyone knows, all microwaves are different, so times may vary. Add salt or other seasonings to taste. *Note:* For macaroni and cheese, I add the cheese sauce to 2 cups of cooked kamut spirals (Types O and A only), but I'm sure other pastas would work equally well. You can also use it to liven up broccoli, asparagus, or other vegetables. *Serves 2.*

PEANUT DRESSING

HIGHLY BENEFICIAL	A, AB	NEUTRAL		AVOID	O, B

½ cup crunchy peanut butter
1 tablespoon honey

¼ cup water
pinch of salt (if using unsalted peanut butter)

Combine all ingredients in a saucepan over low heat, and stir to
mix well. A little more water can be added to thin the sauce if
you choose. Serve warm over noodles or on chicken.
Makes ¾ cup.

TAHINI DRESSING

HIGHLY BENEFICIAL		NEUTRAL	O, A	AVOID	B, AB

Thick and creamy, sesame butter is used in a number of Middle
Eastern dishes such as hummus. Try it on fruit salads.

½ cup tahini
1 tablespoon honey
1 to 2 tablespoons water (or more as needed)

Combine all ingredients in a small bowl and stir until blended.
Drizzle over fruit.   *Makes ¾ cup.*

TOFU-MISO DRESSING

HIGHLY BENEFICIAL	A, AB	NEUTRAL	O	AVOID	B

A savory dressing for rice or vegetables.

½ cake tofu
1 tablespoon miso
2 to 3 tablespoons vegetable stock
2 tablespoons sesame seeds (Type AB omit)

🍴 CYBER RECIPE 🍴

RAW ENZYME RELISH

AUTHOR: Belinda (AeonHealth@aol.com)

TYPE A

A raw enzyme dish to boost digestion. Texture, color, sweet/sour—gets those juices flowing for those As out there!

1 lb. fresh cranberries, cleaned/spun dry
2 cups raw pumpkin seeds
1 large Fuji apple (tart/crisp), unpeeled, diced, and
tossed with lemon juice to prevent discoloration
½ cup diced raw pineapple
½ cup thinly sliced celery
¼ cup plain yogurt
¼ cup blackstrap molasses (or maple syrup)
¾ cup raw cane sugar
3 tablespoons lemon juice
dash fresh finely grated ginger
poppy seeds — small handful
dash allspice
dash cinnamon
dash tarragon
dash salt

In food processor, coarsely chop cranberries and pumpkin seeds. In a large bowl, combine cranberry/seed mixture with fuji apple, raw pineapple, celery, yogurt, blackstrap molasses, raw cane sugar, and lemon juice. Sprinkle with grated ginger, poppy seeds, allspice, cinnamon, tiny pinch of tarragon, and salt. *Serves 12.*

Combine all ingredients in a blender and purée until smooth.
Makes about 1½ cups.

TOFU-PARSLEY DRESSING

HIGHLY BENEFICIAL	A, AB	NEUTRAL	O	AVOID	B

This dressing is delicious over brown rice, with a simple vegetable stir-fry. Try it instead of mayonnaise on a sandwich.

½ cake tofu
2 to 3 tablespoons fresh parsley
2 tablespoons lemon juice
2 teaspoons miso

Combine all ingredients in a blender and purée a few seconds until smooth. This dressing will stay fresh for a few days and will get thicker if allowed to sit.   *Makes 1½ cups.*

SESAME-SEED DRESSING

HIGHLY BENEFICIAL		NEUTRAL	O, A	AVOID	B, AB

This light, creamy dressing is coarser than tahini. Although the sesame seeds are ground with a mortar and pestle, they should not be ground too finely.

4 tablespoons sesame seeds
2 teaspoons soy sauce
3 tablespoons vegetable stock
1 to 2 teaspoons sugar

Toast the sesame seeds briefly, then grind them by hand until crushed but not too pasty. Add soy sauce, stock, and sugar. Continue to grind until a little smoother. *Makes about 1½ cups.*

BASIL PESTO

HIGHLY BENEFICIAL	O, AB	NEUTRAL	A, B	AVOID	

This pesto has no Parmesan cheese and substitutes walnuts for the traditional pignoli nuts. Make it with a mortar and pestle so that the pesto doesn't become too homogenized. A little coarser is better with this pesto. The proportions for the ingredients are approximate, allowing for personal taste.

1 teaspoon coarse salt
½ cup fresh basil
½ cup fresh parsley
2 to 3 cloves garlic, crushed and peeled
½ cup broken walnuts
olive oil

Place salt in mortar and begin adding basil and parsley leaves. Add some garlic, continuing to work in each new addition. Add broken nuts, more leaves, then garlic, until mixture is well ground but not too smooth. Add olive oil slowly, stirring until desired consistency is reached. *Makes about 2 cups.*

CILANTRO PESTO

HIGHLY BENEFICIAL	O, AB	NEUTRAL	A, B	AVOID	

Like basil pesto, this is best made with mortar and pestle. Try it on pasta, rice, or sandwiches. Stir a tablespoon into soup just before serving.

1 teaspoon coarse salt
1 cup fresh cilantro
¼ cup fresh parsley
3 cloves garlic, crushed and peeled
½ cup broken walnuts
olive oil

Place salt in mortar and alternately add cilantro, parsley, garlic, and nuts, incorporating each new addition thoroughly. When you have a coarse paste, slowly add olive oil until you reach the desired consistency. *Makes about 2 cups.*

LEMON-HONEY DRESSING

HIGHLY BENEFICIAL	A, AB	NEUTRAL	O, B	AVOID	

This is a good marinade for fish, and a sweet and tart dressing for salads.

juice of 2 lemons
¼ cup olive oil
1 to 2 tablespoons honey
1 to 2 teaspoons tamari

Combine all ingredients in a jar, seal tightly, and shake well. Season to taste. *Makes 1 cup.*

SEAWEED DRESSING

HIGHLY BENEFICIAL	O	NEUTRAL	A, B, AB	AVOID	

The possibilities for this dressing are endless. Try it on green salads, use it as a dip with fresh green beans and carrot sticks, or toss with rice spaghetti and serve as a cold lunch. This is a good opportunity to use the ends of nori when cracked or torn. Since sea-weed is so expensive, it shouldn't be wasted.

1 cup dulse flakes, or wakame, or nori seaweed
½ cup olive oil
¼ cup sesame seeds (TYPE B AND TYPE AB SUBSTITUTE WALNUTS)
1 tablespoon sesame oil (TYPES A, B, AND AB
SUBSTITUTE OLIVE OIL)
1 teaspoon rice vinegar (TYPE O AND TYPE A AVOID)
1 teaspoon soy sauce
¼ cup water (approximately)

Combine all ingredients in blender and purée, thinning with water until desired consistency is achieved. *Makes 2 cups.*

OLIVE OIL & LEMON DRESSING

HIGHLY BENEFICIAL	O, A, B, AB	NEUTRAL		AVOID	

A basic dressing that should be a staple in every household.

½ cup extra-virgin olive oil
juice of 2 lemons
½ teaspoon dry mustard
½ teaspoon salt
¼ teaspoon honey

Combine all ingredients in a small bowl and whisk until blended. Serve on any salad. *Makes about ¾ cup.*

SWEET VIDALIA ONION DRESSING

HIGHLY BENEFICIAL	O, A, B, AB NEUTRAL		AVOID	

The Vidalia onion is wonderfully sweet and mild. Joined with the tart lemon juice and green parsley, it makes a great accompaniment to mesclun or other mixed green salads.

½ small Vidalia onion
juice of 2 lemons
1 tablespoon chopped fresh parsley
1 teaspoon salt
½ teaspoon sugar
1½ cups olive oil

Grate or finely chop onion. Combine onion and remaining ingredients except oil in a small bowl and allow to marinate 1 hour. After an hour, drizzle oil into onion and lemon mixture and whisk. If dressing separates, shake or whisk again.
Makes about 2 cups.

BALSAMIC MUSTARD VINAIGRETTE

HIGHLY BENEFICIAL		NEUTRAL B, AB	AVOID A, O

A slightly sweet and very satisfying salad dressing.

2 tablespoons honey
2 tablespoons Dijon mustard
½ cup balsamic vinegar
1 cup olive oil

In a food processor, combine honey, mustard, and vinegar. With machine running, slowly drizzle in oil so that it is completely incorporated. This can last in the refrigerator indefinitely. *Makes about 2 cups.*

CUCUMBER-YOGURT SAUCE

HIGHLY BENEFICIAL	B, AB	NEUTRAL	A	AVOID	O

This sauce is ideal with curries; with cold, sliced lamb; and with fresh vegetables for dipping.

2 cups plain yogurt
½ red onion, diced small
1 tablespoon chopped fresh mint
1 tablespoon chopped cilantro
1 small cucumber, peeled, seeded, and diced
2 teaspoons ground cumin
squeeze of lemon juice

Combine all ingredients in a blender and purée until smooth. *Makes about 3 cups.*

PINEAPPLE CHUTNEY

HIGHLY BENEFICIAL	A, B, AB	NEUTRAL	O	AVOID	

1 small onion, diced small
2 tablespoons olive or canola oil
1 ripe pineapple, peeled, cored, and chopped small
1-inch piece fresh ginger, peeled and grated
juice of 2 lemons

1 cup brown sugar
¼ cup pineapple juice
½ cup raisins

In a saucepan, cook onion in oil over medium heat until translucent. Add pineapple and ginger and cook a few minutes. Add remaining ingredients and cook down until thick, about 5 minutes. Cool and serve with grilled tempeh or curried tofu. *Makes about 1 to 1½ quarts.*

PINEAPPLE CHUTNEY–YOGURT SAUCE

HIGHLY BENEFICIAL	A, B, AB	NEUTRAL		AVOID	O

1 cup Pineapple Chutney
2 tablespoons plain yogurt
2 tablespoons canola or commercial mayonnaise

Combine all ingredients in a blender or food processor and purée until smooth. *Makes about 1½ cups.*

FRESH MANGO AND MINT SAUCE

HIGHLY BENEFICIAL		NEUTRAL	O, B	AVOID	A, AB

Serve this sauce over fish, topped with sliced or small whole mint leaves.

1 ripe mango, peeled and pitted
½-inch piece fresh ginger, peeled
juice of 1 lime
2 tablespoons extra-virgin olive oil

1 teaspoon salt
zest of 1 lime
2 tablespoons fresh mint, rolled together, then sliced finely

In a food processor or blender, combine mango, ginger, and lime juice and purée until smooth. While still blending, drizzle in oil. Transfer to bowl. Stir in salt, zest, and mint.
Makes about 1⅓ cups.

HOMEMADE KETCHUP

HIGHLY BENEFICIAL		NEUTRAL	O, AB	AVOID	A, B

This is an interesting variation on ketchup that tastes nothing like the commercial kind in the squeeze bottles.

¾ cup water
⅓ cup tomato paste
2 tablespoons lemon juice
2 tablespoons honey
1 teaspoon tamari sauce

In a small bowl, combine all ingredients, and stir until well blended. *Makes about 1½ cups.*

PEANUT BUTTER SAUCE (GADO-GADO)

HIGHLY BENEFICIAL	A, B, AB	NEUTRAL		AVOID	O

This sauce is a staple for those who love and can eat peanuts. It's versatile enough to use as a dip for vegetables and crackers, as a sauce for fish destined for the broiler, but, above all, as a perfect accompaniment to tempeh and tofu. Double the recipe and keep it in the refrigerator. It lasts a good ten days, if not longer.

1 clove garlic, crushed and peeled
2 scallions
¼ cup coarsely chopped fresh cilantro
½ cup peanut butter
¼ cup tamari sauce
2 tablespoons lemon juice
½ cup water
1 teaspoon peeled and chopped fresh ginger

In a food processor, chop garlic, scallion, and cilantro. Add peanut butter, tamari, and lemon juice and pulse until blended, scraping down bowl as necessary. The mixture will be very thick. With machine running, slowly add some water until desired consistency is reached. *Makes about 2 cups.*

TAHINI SAUCE

HIGHLY BENEFICIAL		NEUTRAL	O, A	AVOID	B, AB

1 clove garlic, crushed slightly and peeled
juice of 1 lime
1-inch piece fresh ginger, peeled and cut in half
¼ cup sesame tahini
½ teaspoon red pepper flakes
1 tablespoon toasted sesame seeds
½ to ¾ cup hot water

Combine all ingredients in the bowl of a food processor or blender. With machine running, slowly add hot water until desired consistency is achieved. *Makes 1 cup.*

FRESH MINT SAUCE

HIGHLY BENEFICIAL		NEUTRAL	B, AB	AVOID	O, A

This is a very versatile recipe that can be used for salads, grilled meats, curried dishes, and fish. It's especially handy if you grow mint, since the recipe calls for a large handful. Double the recipe, and it can hold in the refrigerator for up to two weeks.

1 cup fresh mint leaves, cleaned and dried
½-inch piece fresh ginger, peeled and cut in quarters
1 scallion
3 stalks lemongrass, bottom quarter cut and peeled to soft layer
(reserve tough outer leaves for broth)
1 tablespoon rice wine
1 teaspoon brown rice vinegar
juice of 1 lime
½ teaspoon sugar
¼ cup olive oil

In a blender or food processor, combine all the ingredients, except olive oil and purée. Slowly drizzle oil into the mixture, and blend 10 seconds. Chill thoroughly and serve.
Makes about 1½ cups.

CRANBERRY–HONEY MUSTARD SAUCE

HIGHLY BENEFICIAL		NEUTRAL	O, A, B, AB	AVOID	

This isn't only a sauce. It's also a delicious glaze for roasted poultry, especially turkey. It doesn't work as well on the grill, though.

The sugar in the cranberry jam and honey quickly burns on the open flame.

1 jar all-fruit cranberry jam
2 tablespoons honey
2 tablespoons Dijon mustard
1 clove garlic, crushed and peeled

Combine all ingredients in a small bowl and whisk until blended. Brush on boneless chicken, turkey breast, whole chicken, turkey, or tempeh, and bake in a preheated 350-degree F oven for required amount of time. *Makes about 1½ cups.*

LIME DRESSING

HIGHLY BENEFICIAL		NEUTRAL	O, A, B, AB	AVOID	

A very tasty dressing for mixed greens that is also delicious on fish. The canola oil can be replaced entirely with olive oil in this recipe.

½ teaspoon Garlic-Shallot Mixture (see page 334),
or 2 shallots, finely chopped
2 teaspoons dry mustard
juice and zest from 2 limes
½ teaspoon salt
1 cup canola oil or olive oil

Combine Garlic-Shallot Mixture or 2 shallots, mustard, lime juice, zest, and salt in a small bowl. While whisking briskly, drizzle the oil in a steady stream until it has all been incorporated. For a smoother dressing, use a blender. *Makes 1½ to 2 cups.*

GARLIC-SHALLOT MIXTURE

HIGHLY BENEFICIAL	O, A, AB	NEUTRAL	B	AVOID	

This recipe cuts down on both preparation and cooking time! There are so many recipes that call for chopped garlic, or onions, or both. This is a terrific substitute. Spoon a teaspoon or so into any dish that you're making.

10 cloves garlic, peeled
10 shallots, peeled
olive oil to cover

In a food processor or blender, combine garlic and shallots and pulse on and off, scraping down sides of bowl as necessary, until finely chopped. When desired consistency is reached, transfer to an airtight container and cover with oil. This will be good, refrigerated, for about 10 days or longer.

WILD MUSHROOM SAUCE

HIGHLY BENEFICIAL		NEUTRAL	O, A, B, AB	AVOID	

Any mushroom is suitable for this sauce, but wild mushrooms produce the deepest, most intense flavors as well as a velvety texture. They complement grilled meats, sautéed chicken breasts, or steamed tempeh. Serve this sauce over pasta or almost any grain.

4 tablespoons butter, canola-oil margarine, or olive oil
3 tablespoons Garlic-Shallot Mixture (see page 334)

2 large Portobello mushrooms, stems trimmed, but
not discarded, and sliced
8 oz. tree oyster mushrooms
2 oz. enoki mushrooms (TYPE A OMIT)
2 tablespoons spelt flour
2 tablespoons melted butter or canola-oil margarine
or olive oil
1½ to 2 cups vegetable stock, warmed
¼ cup sherry
salt

Heat 2 tablespoons butter, margarine, or oil. Add Garlic-Shallot
Mixture and sauté for 2 minutes. Add all of the mushrooms
and cook until soft, about 5 minutes. Remove from heat and
set aside. In a separate pan, make a roux, by heating the flour
and browning it ever so slightly. Add the second 2 tablespoons
melted butter or margarine or oil and whisk with the browned
flour until thoroughly blended. It will probably be a bit thick,
but whisk and stir 2 minutes. Slowly add 1 cup warm stock, a
bit at a time, whisking constantly to prevent lumps. Reserve
½ cup to add later, if sauce becomes too thick. Should you add
the stock all at once, the sauce will be lumpy. Slowly pour in a
little at a time. Simmer sauce 5 minutes, and it will thicken.
Add mushrooms, and whatever liquid they have thrown off,
and sherry, and cook over low heat 10 minutes more. If sauce
is too thick, add more stock, again a little at a time, and cook 5
minutes longer. Season to taste with salt and serve hot with
broiled, grilled, or sautéed meats. Try this sauce with tempeh,
tofu, or served over grains or pasta.   *Makes about 3 cups.*

DIPPING SAUCE

HIGHLY BENEFICIAL		NEUTRAL	O, A, B, AB	AVOID	

Use as a dip or marinade for tempeh, fish, or meats.

¼ cup tamari sauce
juice of 1 lime
1 tablespoon sesame oil (TYPE O ONLY) *or olive oil*
2 tablespoons chopped fresh cilantro
1 tablespoon sugar
2 tablespoons brown rice vinegar, or 2 tablespoons lemon juice
1 clove garlic, crushed and peeled

Combine all ingredients in a small bowl. For a great marinade, just add an additional ½ cup olive oil. *Makes about 1 cup.*

MANGO-GINGER CHUTNEY

HIGHLY BENEFICIAL		NEUTRAL	O, B	AVOID	A, AB

This is a quick and simple chutney that goes well with all curry dishes. It is also good with tempeh, fish, and meats, such as lamb.

2 ripe mangoes, peeled and diced
2-inch piece fresh ginger, peeled and grated
4 scallions, sliced
1 teaspoon ground cumin
3 apricots, pitted and sliced
juice of 1 lemon
1 tablespoon brown sugar
2 tablespoons canola or olive oil

Combine all ingredients in a nonreactive saucepan and cook over low heat 15 minutes. Cool and chill. Serve cold.
Makes 2 to 3 cups.

CHUTNEY-YOGURT MAYONNAISE

HIGHLY BENEFICIAL	AB	NEUTRAL	A	AVOID	O, B

This is a perfect dip for grilled chicken, fresh vegetables, or crunchy rice crackers. Try it as an unusual sandwich spread for chicken or fresh grilled tuna.

½ cup plain yogurt
⅓ cup homemade canola- or Olive-Oil Mayonnaise
(see page 318)
3 tablespoons Pineapple Chutney (page 328)
1 teaspoon ground cumin

Combine all ingredients in a small bowl and stir until blended. Cover and chill. Gets even better after a few hours.
Makes about 1 cup.

NANNY MOSKO'S RED PEPPER RELISH

HIGHLY BENEFICIAL	B	NEUTRAL		AVOID	O, A, AB

A long-standing favorite from Martha D'Adamo's family recipe files.

12 red peppers
12 green peppers
12 large onions
3 cups sugar

3 tablespoons salt
1 pint white vinegar

Seed peppers and cut into medium-size pieces; peel and cut onions. In a blender or food processor, chop vegetables by pulsing on and off several seconds, until desired consistency is achieved. Transfer mixture to a large stainless-steel pot. In a mixing bowl, dissolve the sugar and salt in the vinegar. Pour this over the chopped peppers and onions and bring mixture to a boil. Reduce heat and simmer 30 minutes, or until relish begins to thicken. Pour into hot sterile jars, cap, and seal. *Makes 6 to 8 quarts.*

NANNY MOSKO'S BREAD AND BUTTER PICKLES

HIGHLY BENEFICIAL	B	NEUTRAL		AVOID	O, A, AB

These delicious pickles are also from the Martha D'Adamo family files. This is her grandmother's recipe. A great way to pickle some of those delicious garden-fresh cucumbers at the end of the season.

4 quarts sliced cucumbers
4 quarts sliced onions
½ cup salt
3½ cups white vinegar
2 cups sugar
2 teaspoons mustard seeds
2 teaspoons celery seeds
1 teaspoon ground tumeric

Cover cucumbers and onions with salt. Mix well and let stand about 3 hours. In a large nonreactive stockpot, bring the vinegar, sugar, mustard seeds, celery seeds, and turmeric to a boil.

Drain and dry vegetables, then add to the boiling vinegar mixture. Cook 15 minutes. Pack in hot sterile jars, cap, and seal. *Makes about 8 quarts.*

WALNUT-OIL DRESSING

HIGHLY BENEFICIAL	O, AB	NEUTRAL	A	AVOID	B

Enjoy this intensely flavored dressing.

½ cup olive oil
¼ cup walnut oil
2 tablespoons fresh lemon juice
½ teaspoon dry mustard
¼ teaspoon salt
¼ cup walnuts
2 tablespoons chopped fresh parsley

Combine all ingredients in a blender and mix for a minute or two until walnuts are coarsely chopped. Serve over mixed greens. *Makes 1½ cups.*

PLUM BARBECUE SAUCE

HIGHLY BENEFICIAL	O, A, B, AB	NEUTRAL	AVOID	

This piquant plum sauce is on every blood type's Highly Beneficial list! Delicious on chicken and fish, especially a rich tuna steak. If you try to grill with this, it will burn, so reserve for the last few minutes of cooking or serve it on the side.

6 oz. all-fruit plum jam
2 oz. pineapple juice

3 tablespoons tamari sauce
2 cloves garlic, put through a press
2 scallions, thinly sliced
2-inch piece fresh ginger, grated

Combine all ingredients in a small bowl and stir until blended.
Good coarse or smooth. Blend to the consistency you desire.
Makes 1½ cups.

SIMPLE MARINADE

HIGHLY BENEFICIAL	A, AB	NEUTRAL	O, B	AVOID	

This marinade works on chicken, meat, tempeh, or tofu. Also
good on bluefish or mackerel.

3 tablespoons olive oil
2 tablespoons tamari sauce
2 tablespoons Garlic-Shallot Mixture (see page 334)
2 tablespoons chopped fresh cilantro
2 tablespoons lemon juice

Combine all the ingredients in a small bowl and stir. This marinade will hold in the refrigerator for several weeks.
Makes ¾ cup.

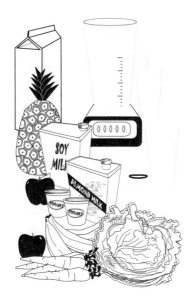

NINETEEN

Beverages

$\mathcal{I}$T DIDN'T TAKE HUMAN BEINGS TOO LONG TO LEARN that there was more to drink than just water. Observing the creatures of the wild, curiosity, accidents of nature, and dire necessity quickly led to the consumption of a vast number of juices, fermented fruit and vegetable potables, and herbal concoctions. Within a relative speck of time, crude beers, wines, and liquors were abundant—and often safer to drink than water. There was no sanitation, and water sources often became quickly fouled and dangerous for consumption.

Today there are countless varieties of waters, juices, milks, sodas, beers, wines, liquors, coffees, teas, and tonics available wherever you go. Perhaps because of this abundance, and the emphasis on "fun" drinks, we have moved away from the idea of beverages as an essential part of a nutritionally sound diet. To underscore this point, many beverages that are considered nutritious are notably vile-tasting, as if anything healthy is necessarily unpleasant and somewhat noxious. The following recipes will dispel that notion entirely. Here are a few suggestions for some interesting drinks you can prepare at home. There are recipes for blender drinks, herbal teas, fresh fruit and vegetable juices, and some favorite beverage choices from around the world.

In many instances, these recipes offer protein- and fruit-rich drinks that can provide nutritious between-meal snacks for adults as well as ideal tide-me-overs for hungry children just home from school. Many of the recipes also offer substantial nourishment for those who otherwise might not be able to consume a more complex meal because of age or infirmity.

Yogurt Drinks

TYPE A, TYPE B, AND TYPE AB can eat cow, goat, or sheep milk–based yogurt. Although sheep's milk yogurt is probably the least commercially available, its texture and richness are unparalleled. Nonetheless, there are a lot of very good commercial yogurts available. *Kefir* is whole or partially skimmed milk that has been fermented until it has a slightly fizzy, tangier taste than yogurt. *Kefir* is a very popular drink in eastern Europe, India, and the Middle East. *Laban*, a thicker version of yogurt, is widely used for cooking as well.

PINEAPPLE SMOOTHIE

HIGHLY BENEFICIAL	A, B, AB	NEUTRAL		AVOID	O

1 cup yogurt
1 cup chopped pineapple
½ cup pineapple juice
fresh mint leaves

Combine yogurt, pineapple, and pineapple juice in a blender and blend well until smooth. Pour into tall glass and garnish with mint leaves.

APRICOT SMOOTHIE

HIGHLY BENEFICIAL	A, B, AB	NEUTRAL		AVOID	O

1 cup yogurt
1 cup fresh apricots
½ cup apricot juice

Combine all ingredients in a blender and blend until smooth. *Serves 1 or 2.*

BANANA SMOOTHIE

HIGHLY BENEFICIAL	B	NEUTRAL		AVOID	O, A, AB

1 cup yogurt
1 large, ripe banana, cut into chunks
½ cup pineapple juice

Combine all ingredients in a blender and blend until smooth. *Serves 1 or 2.*

MINT SMOOTHIE

HIGHLY BENEFICIAL	B, AB	NEUTRAL	A	AVOID	O

1 cup yogurt
¼ cup fresh mint

1 cup water
½ teaspoon ground, roasted cumin seeds
sprinkle of salt

Combine all ingredients in a blender and blend until smooth. Drink ice cold.   *Serves 1.*

———————

ROSE-WATER LASSI

HIGHLY BENEFICIAL	B, AB	NEUTRAL	A	AVOID	O

This is a classic Indian lassi. Serve it ice cold. Type A and Type AB can use a low-fat yogurt.

1 cup whole-milk yogurt
2 teaspoons rose water
3 tablespoons sugar

Combine all ingredients in a blender and blend until smooth. *Serves 1.*

Soy Beverages

SOY MILK is a fabulous alternative to dairy for Type O and Type A. Soy milk is also well tolerated by Type B and Type AB. This places soy milk in the rare position of being good for all blood types! It isn't really enough to tell you to just go out and buy some soy milk, because in just the last few years the field of manufacturers has broadened considerably. Not only that, but there's whole soy milk, nonfat soy milk, 1% low-fat soy milk, soy drink, and plain, vanilla-, or cocoa-flavored soy milks and beverages. Be sure to check the ingredients of soy and rice milks because brands vary. Some use barley malt sweeteners (avoid for Type B) and oils.

For a pleasing taste and texture, try a blend of soy milk and brown rice milk. The blend is smooth and rich, while relatively low in fat and calories. Many people initially dislike the taste and texture of soy milk. Depending on the mixture and the brand, soy milk can vary in consistency and taste, so experiment until you find the brand you like. These fruit smoothies are one of the best ways to enjoy soy milk.

MANGO-LIME SMOOTHIE

HIGHLY BENEFICIAL		NEUTRAL	O, B	AVOID	A, AB

1 cup soy milk
1 ripe mango, peeled, pitted and cut into chunks
½ cup pineapple juice
juice of ½ lime

Combine all ingredients in a blender and blend until smooth. Serve very cold. *Serves 1 or 2.*

PAPAYA-KIWI SMOOTHIE

HIGHLY BENEFICIAL	AB	NEUTRAL	O, B	AVOID	A

1 cup soy milk
½ small papaya, peeled, seeded and cut into chunks
1 kiwi, peeled and cut into chunks
½ cup papaya juice

Combine all ingredients in a blender and blend until smooth. Serve very cold. *Serves 1.*

CHERRY-PEACH SMOOTHIE

HIGHLY BENEFICIAL	A, AB	NEUTRAL	O, B	AVOID	

1 cup soy milk
½ cup black cherries, pitted
2 ripe peaches, pitted and cut into chunks
1 cup cherry juice

Combine all ingredients in a blender and blend until smooth.
Serve ice cold.   *Serves 2.*

BANANA-PAPAYA SMOOTHIE

HIGHLY BENEFICIAL		NEUTRAL	O, B	AVOID	A, AB

A rich and delicious tropical treat!

1 cup soy milk
1 ripe banana, cut into chunks
½ ripe papaya, peeled, seeded, and cut into chunks
½ cup pineapple juice

Combine all ingredients in a blender and blend until smooth.
Drink well chilled.   *Serves 2.*

DATE-PRUNE SMOOTHIE

HIGHLY BENEFICIAL	A	NEUTRAL	O, B, AB	AVOID	

Rich, delicious, and incredibly good for you. If it's too rich, you can always blend in a few ice cubes to thin its consistency, while making it ice cold.

1 cup soy milk
4 pitted prunes
2 to 3 pitted dates
1 cup prune juice

Combine all ingredients in a blender and blend until smooth. Enjoy ice cold. *Serves 2.*

GRAPE-PEACH SMOOTHIE

HIGHLY BENEFICIAL		NEUTRAL	O, A, B, AB	AVOID	

Light, sweet, and tart, depending on the variety of grape and the amount of lime juice you use.

½ cup soy milk
½ cup apple juice
1 small peach, peeled, pitted, and cut into chunks
½ cup of seedless grapes
juice of ½ lime

Combine all ingredients in a blender. Blend thoroughly and enjoy. *Serves 1.*

SILKEN TOFU SMOOTHIE

HIGHLY BENEFICIAL	A, AB	NEUTRAL	O	AVOID	B

Instead of soy milk, this recipe calls for the smoothest, most custardlike tofu—silken tofu. It may help you to start overcoming any aversions you may have to tofu.

1 cup fresh pineapple chunks
3 oz. silken tofu
½ cup pineapple juice
1 fresh apricot, peeled and pitted
4 ice cubes

Combine all ingredients in a blender and mix 2 minutes, or until smooth. Drink immediately.   *Serves 1 to 2.*

Rice Milk

HIGHLY BENEFICIAL		NEUTRAL	O, A, B, AB	AVOID	

LESS COMMONLY used than soy milk, rice milk—not an actual milk, of course—is another excellent alternative to dairy. Rice milk is much lighter and sweeter than soy milk. It also has the advantage of being perfectly assimilable by all blood types. It can be used as an alternative to soy milk or yogurt in all of the suggested blender recipes, poured over cereal, or it can simply be enjoyed as a refreshing beverage. Be sure to check the ingredients. Some brands use safflower oil, which all blood types should avoid; and canola oil, which Type Bs should avoid.

Rice milk makes a thinner shake than either soy milk or yogurt. It is available fortified with calcium, a real benefit for Type O. Use it as you would either yogurt or soy milk.

Almond Milk and Oat Milk

HIGHLY BENEFICIAL		NEUTRAL	O, A, B, AB	AVOID	

ALMOND AND OAT MILK are yet two more alternatives to dairy-based products and are interesting and delightful in their own right. Check the ingredients, as some brands use barley malt, which Type B and Type AB should avoid. Use them as the base for shakes, pour over cereals, or drink them straight, ice cold.

Fruit and Vegetable Juices

THERE IS SUCH a wide variety of high-quality fruit and vegetable juices available that it seems foolish to place any caveats on their use. They can be tremendously valuable sources of nutrition. But, please, if you buy juice commercially, check the label. So many juices today contain only a fraction of concentrated juice and an enormous amount of water and cheap sweetener, usually corn syrup.

As many people have discovered over the years, owning a juicer can make "eating" your fruits and vegetables a whole new experience. All of the directions for preparation of these juices are the same: Clean the produce thoroughly, place it in the juicer, and enjoy!

CARROT-CELERY JUICE

HIGHLY BENEFICIAL	A, B, AB	NEUTRAL	O	AVOID	

Carrot juice can be very sweet, so add more celery if you prefer a lighter juice. Celery contains a good amount of sodium, so it balances the sweetness of the carrot.

4 washed carrots, ends removed
2 washed stalks celery, leaves on

Serves 1 to 2.

CARROT-GINGER JUICE

HIGHLY BENEFICIAL	A, AB	NEUTRAL	O, B	AVOID	

This can be a spicy drink, so add ginger in small amounts.

4 washed carrots, ends removed
½- to 1-inch piece fresh ginger, or to taste

Serves 1 to 2.

CARROT-CUCUMBER JUICE

HIGHLY BENEFICIAL	A, AB	NEUTRAL	O, B	AVOID	

A light and refreshing drink. The cucumber and carrot are a surprisingly delicate combination.

4 washed carrots, ends removed
1 cucumber, peeled if not organic

Serves 1 to 2.

CARROT-APPLE JUICE

HIGHLY BENEFICIAL		NEUTRAL	O, A, B, AB	AVOID	

This is a seductive combination of vegetable and fruit, both sweet and delicious.

4 washed carrots, ends removed
1 apple, peeled if not organic

Serves 1 to 2.

APPLE-GRAPE JUICE

HIGHLY BENEFICIAL		NEUTRAL	O, A, B, AB	AVOID	

3 apples, peeled if not organic
1 cluster of washed grapes, stems removed

Serves 1 to 2.

Herbal Teas

HERBAL TEAS can be far more than a comforting, relaxing infusion. Many of the known folk medicines of the world can be found sitting on a health-food or supermarket shelf, neatly packaged and labeled. Fatigue, depression, malaise, indigestion, constipation, headaches, and much more can be treated with a cup or two of the right herbal tea. There is an entire potent world within our reach. As we detailed for you elsewhere, there are many herbal concoctions that are ideal for each of the different blood types.

🍴 CYBER RECIPE 🍴

GREEN TEA–LIME SLUSHIE
AUTHOR: Belinda (AeonHealth@aol.com)

TYPES A, B, AB

Drink this instead of a Lime and Rum Slush. Helps your digestion.

¼ cup maple syrup (sweeten more to taste)
1 quart brewed hot green tea
pinch of cinnamon (TYPE B CAN AVOID)
pinch of tarragon
pinch of ginger
juice of 2 limes, including pulp
2 teaspoons lime zest

Add syrup to hot tea and mix. Add spices. Add remaining ingredients (saving 1 teaspoon lime zest for garnish). Freeze mixture in ice trays.

To serve: Run frozen tea through blender or juicer until consistency of slush. Pour into individual serving glasses and garnish with lime slices and zest curls.   *Serves 2 to 4.*

TWENTY

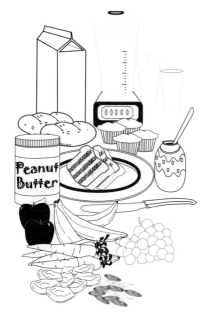

Snacks, Treats, & Munchies

$\mathcal{S}$NACKS ARE BY NO MEANS ESSENTIAL TO GOOD EATING. But let's face the facts: They're here to stay, especially if you have kids. Why not give them a healthy boost? Rather than letting children fill up on the highly processed junk foods that are heavily advertised to appeal to kids, making a little extra effort can provide some delightful alternatives.

Snacks for kids should be quick, easy, and on hand. Whatever you choose not only has to satisfy between-meal hunger, but also has to provide a good, nutritious boost to their systems. Snacks should be something older kids can serve themselves. Healthy snacks can be on the kitchen table, ready to eat, a few minutes after the kids walk in the door from school or play.

Trail Mix

ORIGINALLY A high-calorie energy sustainer for extended hiking, trail mix started becoming very popular in the late 1960s. Affectionately nicknamed Gorp, the basic recipe has been modified to suit the different blood types. Ingredients for trail mix can be adjusted according to your taste. It is made primarily of nuts, seeds, and dried fruits, which are concentrated energy sources, so a little trail mix goes a long way. For school, in the car, or on a hike, trail mix may be one of the most satisfying treats ever invented. The crunch of the nuts and seeds and the intense sweetness of the dried fruits combine to provide a filling, satisfying combination. Trail mix is very simple to prepare. The following recipes provide three variations of the basic mix for each of the four blood types. Merely combine all ingredients and store in a tightly covered glass container.

Type O Trail Mixes

TYPE O TRAIL MIX #1

1 cup walnuts, broken into pieces
½ cup filberts, halved
½ cup dried apricots, quartered
½ cup dried cherries
½ cup dairy-free semisweet chocolate or carob chips

TYPE O TRAIL MIX #2

1 cup pumpkin seeds
½ cup sunflower seeds
½ cup dried pears, chopped
½ cup dried pineapple, chopped

TYPE O TRAIL MIX #3

1 cup dried cranberries
1 cup sunflower seeds
½ cup walnuts, broken into pieces
½ cup dairy-free chocolate chips

Type A Trail Mixes

TYPE A TRAIL MIX #1

1 cup peanuts
½ cup dried apricots, quartered
½ cup raisins

TYPE A TRAIL MIX #2

1 cup pumpkin seeds
½ cup sunflower seeds
½ cup walnuts, broken into pieces
1 cup dried pineapple, chopped

TYPE A TRAIL MIX #3

1 cup almonds, chopped
1 cup dried cherries
½ cup dairy-free semisweet chocolate or carob chips

Type B Trail Mixes

TYPE B TRAIL MIX #1

1 cup Brazil nuts, chopped
½ cup dried bananas, sliced
½ cup dried apricots, quartered

TYPE B TRAIL MIX #2

1 cup macadamia nuts, halved
1 cup dried pineapple, chopped
1 cup dried cranberries

TYPE B TRAIL MIX #3

½ cup pecans, broken into pieces
½ cup almonds, chopped
½ cup raisins
½ cup dried cherries
1 cup semisweet chocolate or carob chips

Type AB Trail Mixes

TYPE AB TRAIL MIX #1

1½ cups peanuts
1 cup walnuts, broken into pieces
½ cup raisins
½ cup dried apricots, quartered

TYPE AB TRAIL MIX #2

½ cup cashews
½ cup toasted pignoli
½ cup dried cranberries

TYPE AB TRAIL MIX #3

½ cup pistachios
1 cup dried cherries
½ cup dried pineapple, chopped
1 cup dairy-free semisweet chocolate or carob chips

All of the trail-mix combinations can be endlessly adjusted and altered, so you need never get bored. Consult your Blood Type lists and take it from there. A final note of caution: Sitting around and watching TV while eating trail mix can be hazardous to your waistline. Remember, nuts, seeds, and dried fruits are not only high in vitamins, minerals, and fiber, they're also high in fat and calories. These mixes are best eaten to sustain energy during performance-oriented activities such as hiking, cycling, or other high calorie–burning sports.

Candies, Toasted Seeds, & Dips

ALMOND-BUTTER CANDY

HIGHLY BENEFICIAL		NEUTRAL	O, A	AVOID	B, AB

1 cup plus 2 tablespoons ground sesame or sunflower seeds
¼ cup dried figs, finely sliced
¼ cup dried apricots, finely sliced
½ cup almond butter
1 to 2 tablespoons honey

Reserve 2 tablespoons sesame or sunflower seeds. Grind the rest of the seeds in a blender until powdery. Sprinkle several tablespoons over dried fruit, and toss to coat and separate the sticky little pieces of fruit. Add remainder of ground seeds to almond butter and stir until blended. Add honey, then dried fruit, blending well with a fork or your hands. Form mixture into balls and roll each one in sesame seeds.
Makes 20 to 24 candies.

PEANUT-BUTTER CANDY

HIGHLY BENEFICIAL	A, AB	NEUTRAL		AVOID	O, B

Without honey this is a delicious but not very sweet candy. Add a tablespoon or more of honey to the recipe as you prepare it, adjusting the sweetness to taste.

1 cup chunky peanut butter
6 tablespoons powdered goat's milk
½ cup dried cherries, halved
½ cup dried apricots, quartered
honey
½ cup walnuts, chopped

Combine peanut butter and 5 tablespoons of the powdered goat's milk in a small bowl and stir until blended. Sprinkle remaining tablespoon of powdered goat's milk over the dried fruit to separate it somewhat. Mix fruit with peanut butter and honey to taste, adding additional powdered milk if necessary for desired consistency. Shape into balls, and roll in the chopped walnuts. *Makes 20 to 24 candies.*

TAMARI-TOASTED SUNFLOWER SEEDS

HIGHLY BENEFICIAL		NEUTRAL	O, A	AVOID	B, AB

4 oz. raw shelled sunflower seeds
1 tablespoon tamari sauce
½ cup of raisins

In a large skillet, heat sunflower seeds over medium heat until almost popping. Flip around to toast evenly, turn off heat, then add tamari. Toss seeds only a few more seconds. The seeds should be well coated, but don't let the tamari burn. Mix with raisins for a sweet and savory snack.   *Serves 2.*

TAMARI-TOASTED PUMPKIN SEEDS

HIGHLY BENEFICIAL	O, A	NEUTRAL		AVOID	B, AB

4 oz. raw pumpkin seeds
1 tablespoon tamari sauce

In a large skillet, heat pumpkin seeds over medium heat until almost popping. Pumpkin seeds behave a lot like popcorn. Shake pan so bottoms of seeds don't burn. Toss a few times, turn off heat, then add tamari. Toss again and cook a few more seconds. Remove seeds from pan and cool.   *Serves 1 to 2.*

Note: This same treatment can be applied to a wide range of nuts as well. Raw cashews, almonds, filberts, peanuts, and Brazil nuts can all be quickly toasted and coated with the salty tamari sauce, according to your blood type.

CURRY DIP

HIGHLY BENEFICIAL		NEUTRAL	O, A, B, AB	AVOID	

Use this spicy dip for fresh vegetables and apples. It also makes an unusual substitute for plain mayonnaise in salads and on sandwiches.

1 cup homemade mayonnaise (see page 318) (TYPE B SHOULD
SUBSTITUTE COMMERCIAL MAYONNAISE)
1 tablespoon lemon juice
1 tablespoon good-quality ground curry powder

1 tablespoon ground cumin
1 tablespoon ground coriander powder
1 tablespoon ground mustard seed

Mix all ingredients together until well blended and serve. Store in a tightly covered glass container.   *Makes about 1½ cups.*

BLACK BEAN DIP

HIGHLY BENEFICIAL	A	NEUTRAL	O	AVOID	B, AB

This dip is very easy to put together and tastes great. If a spicy black bean dip is desired, Type O can add chopped jalapeño peppers or a hot pepper sauce to the basic recipe.

2 cups cooked black beans, or 1 can black beans,
rinsed well and drained
juice of ½ lemon
1 teaspoon salt
½ to 1 cup vegetable stock or water
1 small red onion, diced small
1 tablespoon chopped cilantro

In a food processor or blender, purée beans. Add lemon juice, salt, and a little of the liquid and blend until desired consistency is achieved. Transfer to mixing bowl. Stir in red onion and cilantro. Adjust seasonings and serve chilled with homemade quinoa tortilla chips.   *Makes 4 cups.*

HUMMUS

HIGHLY BENEFICIAL		NEUTRAL	O	AVOID	A, B, AB

The humble chickpea, or garbanzo bean, which is the main ingredient of hummus, has been central to the cuisine of many nations for thousands of years. Ground chickpeas also form the basis for the deep-fried Middle Eastern staple *falafel*. Hummus has many possibilities. Try it as a dip for raw vegetables. It's great as a spread for bread or crackers, as a filling for garden-fresh tomatoes, or even as a delicious sandwich spread. Hummus is quick and easy to make if you use a blender or food processor.

1 can garbanzo beans, drained and rinsed
⅓ cup tahini
juice of 1 small lemon
1 to 2 cloves garlic
½ teaspoon salt
cayenne pepper
2 tablespoons toasted sesame seeds (optional)

Combine all ingredients, except sesame seeds, in blender or food processor and purée until smooth. You may have to turn off the blender and scrape down the sides periodically. If using toasted sesame seeds, heat a heavy skillet over medium heat. Add seeds and shake skillet for a minute or two until seeds begin to pop. Stir them into the puréed hummus with a spoon. Store in a tightly covered glass container.
Makes 2½ cups.

30-Day
Menu Plans:
O, A, B, AB

HEN YOU DECIDED TO FOLLOW THE BLOOD TYPE Diet, you made a very big commitment to change the way you eat and live. But you may still feel some uncertainty about exactly what your meals will look like. These menus offer a road map for your blood type. They show you how to take the food lists and the recipes and organize them into a daily diet that will set you on the path to staying healthy, living longer, and achieving your ideal weight.

Included here is a 30-Day Menu Plan for each blood type. As you grow accustomed to eating right for your type, you'll eventually develop a menu plan of your own. The goal is to reach a stage where it becomes natural for you to eat the foods that are going to do you the most good. Note that beverages are listed with most meals, but I suggest you drink them one half hour before or after eating, rather than with the meal. Be sure to consult *Eat Right 4 Your Type* and chapter 4 of this book to determine the specific requirements of your personal situation—for example, if you need to lose weight, suffer from a medical condition, or have a special susceptibility to disease because of your blood type. Eating well and living well are on the same path.

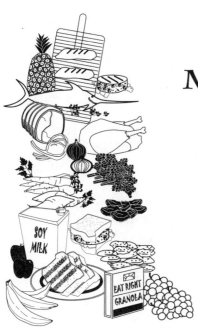

30-Day
Menus for
Type

O

DAY 1

Breakfast
Single-egg omelet with
  grated carrot and
  zucchini
Glass of pineapple juice
Rose hips tea

Snack
2 plums
Glass of soy milk

Lunch
Tuna salad on rye crisps
Iced fenugreek tea

Snack
Carrot-ginger juice

Dinner
Fettuccine with lamb
  sausages
Green salad with honey-
  lemon dressing
Spelt baguette
Glass of wine
Fresh figs

D A Y 2	
Breakfast 1 slice of Ezekiel toast with black cherry preserves Ginger tea	Iced seltzer water Handful of grapes **Snack** Tamari pumpkin seeds
Snack Fresh pineapple Grape juice and seltzer	**Dinner** Roast turkey with sage and rosemary Brown-rice pilaf with carrots and onions Steamed broccoli Seltzer
Lunch Hamburger with melted goat Cheddar and slice of tomato	

D A Y 3	
Breakfast Single-egg omelet with broccoli and rice pilaf Slippery elm tea	**Snack** Handful of walnuts and raisins **Dinner** Grilled whole salmon with basil pesto
Snack ½ grapefruit Glass of soy-rice milk	Grilled sweet potatoes Romaine salad with Caesar dressing Glass of white wine
Lunch Sliced turkey on spelt bread with mayonnaise, lettuce, and tomato Cranberry juice and seltzer	

DAY 4

Breakfast
Silken tofu scramble with
  banana and blueberries
Rose hips tea

Snack
Rice cake with soy butter
  and jam
Green tea

Lunch
Salmon salad with
  mayonnaise and
  chopped fresh dill on a
  bed of greens

Rye Crisps
Iced fenugreek tea

Snack
Pear
Glass of soy milk

Dinner
Rice spaghetti with meat
  sauce
Steamed artichoke
French baguette
Chamomile tea

DAY 5

Breakfast
Poached egg on toasted
  Ezekiel bread
½ grapefruit
Slippery elm tea

Snack
Bananna–silken tofu shake
  with peach juice

Lunch
Turkey vegetable soup
French bread
Glass of seltzer

Snack
Figs with goat cheese and
  walnuts

Dinner
Grilled swordfish with lime
  wedge
Sweet potato salad (from
  leftover grilled sweet
  potatoes)
Grilled red peppers
Glass of white wine

D A Y   6

Breakfast
Wild rice–flour pancakes
   with maple syrup
Fresh berries
Mulberry tea

Snack
Banana–silken tofu shake

Lunch
Quinoa tortilla filled with
   leftover rice, red
   peppers, and romaine,
   served with a tahini
   dressing

Seltzer
2 apricots

Snack
Carrot-ginger juice

Dinner
Curried leg of lamb
Basmati rice
Fresh mango chutney
Spinach salad with grated
   hard-boiled egg
Glass of red wine

D A Y   7

Breakfast
Single-egg omelet with
   fresh spinach and feta
   cheese
Fenugreek tea

Snack
Mixed plums
Ginger tea

Lunch
Sliced cold lamb on a bed
   of romaine with mint
   sauce
Iced rose hips tea

Snack
Carrot sticks and pan-fried
   onion dip

Dinner
Country vegetable stew
   with pinto beans
Wild rice salad
Fresh sliced peaches,
   nectarines, figs, and
   plums
Shortbread

DAY 8

Breakfast
Rice crackers with almond
   and prune butters
Sarsaparilla tea

Snack
Apple with walnuts and
   raisins

Lunch
Grilled turkey burger with
   melted goat Cheddar
Sliced tomato and
   cucumbers

Glass of seltzer and
   pineapple juice

Snack
Banana–soy milk smoothie

Dinner
Stir-fried shrimp with bok
   choy, red pepper,
   broccoli, garlic, onion,
   and tamari sauce
Sushi rice
Iced ginger tea
Fig cookies

DAY 9

Breakfast
Frittata with leftover
   vegetables and rice
Peppermint tea

Snack
Plums and apricots
Prune juice and seltzer

Lunch
Grilled goat Cheddar on
   Ezekiel bread
Iced ginseng tea

Snack
Apple-carrot juice

Dinner
Turkey burritos with
   quinoa tortilla
Rice and black beans
Jicama sticks with
   pineapple salsa
Beer

D A Y   1 0

Breakfast
French toast with sautéed
  blueberries
Rose hips tea

Snack
Banana–soy milk smoothie

Lunch
Cuban black bean soup
Glass of seltzer and cherry
  juice

Snack
Apple and goat Cheddar
  slices with Rye Crisp

Dinner
Grilled liver with Vidalia
  onions
Steamed broccoli with
  dipping sauce
Brown rice pilaf

D A Y   1 1

Breakfast
Fried egg on brown rice
  pilaf
Fenugreek tea

Snack
Banana spelt muffin
Peppermint tea

Lunch
Grilled chicken breast on
  toasted spelt bread with
  lettuce and tomato
Mixed plums
Mineral water

Snack
Tamari pumpkin seeds
Carrot-ginger juice

Dinner
Grilled filet of beef with
  Portobello mushroom
  sauce
Braised leeks
Spinach salad with lemon
  vinaigrette
Glass of red wine
Shortbread

D A Y   1 2

Breakfast
Spinach frittata
Fenugreek tea

Snack
Fresh or dried figs or
   apricots
Glass of seltzer with lemon

Lunch
Curried carrot and ginger
   soup
Lettuce and tomato salad
Prune juice and seltzer

Snack
Walnut cookies
Ginseng tea

Dinner
Pasta with green
   vegetables
Caesar salad
Plum tart
Rose hips tea

D A Y   1 3

Breakfast
Banana-nut muffin
Peppermint tea

Snack
Fresh carrot juice

Lunch
Slices of roast beef with
   pan-fried onion dip
   rolled in a romaine leaf
Pears and walnuts
Mineral water

Snack
Rye Crisps with soy-nut
   butter

Dinner
Braised veal shanks
Onion and fennel confit
Rice
Stir-fried sugar snap peas
Glass of wine

D A Y   1 4

Breakfast
1 poached egg on Ezekiel
  bread
½ grapefruit and sliced
  banana
Mint tea

Snack
Walnuts, raisins, and
  chocolate chips
Mineral water

Lunch
Turkey burger

Lettuce and tomato
Glass of seltzer

Snack
Red pepper strips with
  curry dip
Ginseng tea

Dinner
Indian lamb stew with
  spinach
Basmati rice
Mango chutney
Fenugreek tea

D A Y   1 5

Breakfast
Spelt pancakes with
  blueberry preserves
Sliced bananas
Slippery elm tea

Snack
Trail mix
Mineral water

Lunch
Tuna salad on a bed of
  mesclun
Pineapple juice and seltzer

Snack
Walnut cookies
Peppermint tea

Dinner
Veal stew with fennel
Wild and basmati rice pilaf
Steamed artichokes
Glass of wine

D A Y   1 6

Breakfast
Scrambled eggs with
  Ezekiel toast and
  pineapple preserves
½ grapefruit
Cayenne tea

Snack
Banana–soy milk
  smoothie

Lunch
White bean soup with
  Swiss chard

Rye Crisps with
  goat cheese
Glass of seltzer with lemon

Snack
Banana muffin
Sarsaparilla tea

Dinner
Sautéed monkfish fingers
Sweet potato pancakes
Sesame broccoli
Fenugreek tea

D A Y   1 7

Breakfast
Apricot–silken tofu shake
Rose hips tea
1 slice of millet toast with
  blueberry preserves

Snack
Banana slices spread with
  almond butter
Peppermint tea

Lunch
Cheeseburger (with goat
  Cheddar)

Mesclun salad with
  cucumbers

Snack
2 plums
Ginger tea

Dinner
Roast turkey
Buttered spelt noodles
Applesauce
Steamed peas
Glass of wine

D A Y   1 8

Breakfast
French crêpes with
  sautéed peaches
Rose hips tea

Snack
Pineapple-banana
  smoothie with soy milk

Lunch
Mushroom-barley soup
Mixed lettuces with sliced
  pears and goat cheese
Seltzer with apricot juice

Snack
Carrot sticks with black
  bean dip
Mineral water

Dinner
Broiled bluefish with garlic
  and parsley
Sushi rice
Mixed stir-fried vegetables
Rice wine
  Plum tart

D A Y   1 9

Breakfast
Cherry-almond muffin
Bowl of sliced mixed
  plums and blueberries
Slippery elm tea

Snack
Apple with walnuts and
  goat cheese
Seltzer with lemon

Lunch
Sliced turkey on a bed of
  lettuce

Carrot-raisin salad
Seltzer with black cherry
  juice

Snack
Pecorino romano slices
  with Wasa bread
Dandelion tea

Dinner
Grilled sirloin steak
Cellophane noodles
Braised spinach with garlic
Glass of rice wine

DAY 20

Breakfast
Spelt flakes with raisins
  and soy milk
Banana
Ginger tea

Snack
Rye crackers with cherry
  preserves
Seltzer

Lunch
Salmon salad on romaine
  leaves

Sliced plums
Rose hips tea

Snack
Carrot celery juice

Dinner
Liver with onions
Brown-rice pilaf
Mesclun salad
Glass of wine

DAY 21

Breakfast
1 poached egg
2 slices of apricot-almond
  toast with butter
Ginseng tea

Snack
Apple and banana
Glass of seltzer

Lunch
Gingered squash soup
Rice cracker with soft goat
  cheese

Snack
2 walnut cookies
Peppermint tea

Dinner
Venison stew
Pan-fried sweet potatoes
Braised greens with garlic

D A Y   2 2

Breakfast
Pineapple-banana
 smoothie with soy milk

Snack
English muffin with
 raspberry preserves
Mulberry tea

Lunch
Salmon burgers
Sliced tomato with basil
Carrot juice with ginger

Snack
Sliced apple with almond
 butter
Ginger tea

Dinner
Broiled lamb chops with
 mint sauce
Brown rice
Green been salad with
 walnuts and goat cheese

D A Y   2 3

Breakfast
Blueberry pancakes
Peppermint tea

Snack
Carrots and green beans
 with dip
Mineral water with lemon

Lunch
Simple fish soup
Spelt roll
Seltzer with pineapple
 juice

Snack
2 plums
Iced ginger tea

Dinner
Curried lamb stew with
 mango chutney
Basmati rice
Braised leeks
Fenugreek tea

DAY 24

Breakfast
Quinoa muffin
Fresh figs with goat cheese
Slippery elm tea

Snack
Banana–silken tofu
  smoothie

Lunch
Pinto bean soup
Mesclun salad
Seltzer with lemon

Snack
Walnut cookie
Green tea

Dinner
Tofu-vegetable stir-fry
Brown rice
Fresh sliced mangoes
Glass of red wine

DAY 25

Breakfast
2 scrambled eggs
2 slices of Ezekiel toast
  with grape preserves
Peppermint tea

Snack
Pineapple–soy milk shake

Lunch
Tuna salad with rye
  crackers
Romaine salad
Glass of seltzer

Snack
Bowl of gingered pumpkin
  soup

Dinner
Pan-fried grouper
Sweet potato pancakes
Wilted greens
Fresh sliced fruit
Glass of white wine

D A Y   2 6

Breakfast
Silken tofu scramble with
  sautéed apples or pears
Rose hips tea

Snack
Rice crackers with goat
  cheese
Glass of seltzer

Lunch
Turkey burger with melted
  goat Cheddar
Sliced tomato and romaine
Mineral water

Snack
Apples and walnuts
Herb tea

Dinner
Wild rice soup
1 slice of whole-grain spelt
  bread with apple butter
Arugula salad
Glass of white wine

D A Y   2 7

Breakfast
Banana–soy milk smoothie

Snack
Grapes
Slippery elm tea

Lunch
Chicken salad sandwich
  with lettuce and tomato
  on spelt bread
Seltzer with prune juice

Snack
Apple with goat cheese
Ginger tea

Dinner
Broiled snapper
Penne with broccoli rabe
  and garlic
Fresh fruit
Glass of wine

DAY 28

Breakfast
Single-egg omelet with
  tomato, mozzarella, and
  basil
2 slices of spelt toast with
  apricot preserves
Herb tea

Snack
2 plums
Glass of soy milk

Lunch
Salmon salad on romaine
  leaves
Seltzer with lime

Snack
Fresh figs and apricots
Rose hips tea

Dinner
Turkey cutlets
Spelt noodles
Steamed broccoli with
  lemon
Pineapple slices

DAY 29

Breakfast
2 slices of Ezekiel toast
  with almond butter and
  cherry preserves
Ginseng tea

Snack
Banana–soy milk smoothie

Lunch
Simple fish soup
Tossed salad

Snack
Carrot sticks with curry dip
Green tea

Dinner
Spaghetti and meat sauce
Steamed artichokes
Glass of red wine

D A Y   3 0

Breakfast
Single-egg omelet with
   artichoke hearts,
   broccoli, and goat cheese
1 slice of spelt toast with
   butter
Mulberry tea

Snack
Banana-peach smoothie

Lunch
Greek salad
Seltzer with lemon

Snack
Pear
Raisins and walnuts
Ginger tea

Dinner
Broiled Sole
Green green pasta
Glass of wine
Walnut shortbread

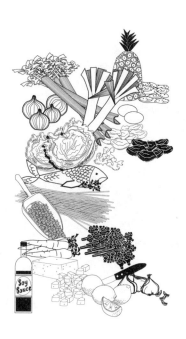

30-Day Menus for Type

A

D A Y 1	
Breakfast Silken tofu scramble with Vidalia onion and broccoli Bowl of blueberries Coffee Glass of water with lemon **Snack** Yogurt with raisins, sunflower seeds, and honey **Lunch** Quinoa-flour tortillas filled with adzuki beans, goat	Cheddar, diced onion, and sprouts Pineapple salsa Iced ginseng tea **Snack** Iced vanilla nut coffee with rice milk **Dinner** Rice spaghetti with stir-fried spinach, carrots, Portobello mushrooms, onion, and garlic ı slice spelt French bread Glass of wine

D A Y   2

Breakfast
Rice cakes with almond
  butter and cherry
  preserves
Rose hips tea

Snack
2 plums
Apricot juice

Lunch
Black bean soup
1 piece of corn bread
Iced burdock tea

Snack
Carrot juice

Dinner
Tofu with peanuts and
  apricots
Brown rice
Steamed spinach

D A Y   3

Breakfast
Buckwheat pancakes with
  blueberry syrup
Toasted almond coffee
  with almond milk

Snack
Fresh pineapple–soy
  milk shake

Lunch
Salad of romaine, grated
  carrot, onion, and flaked
salmon with lime
  vinaigrette
Carrot cucumber juice

Snack
Handful of raisins and
  peanuts

Dinner
Quinoa tortillas with
  black beans
Brown rice
Braised escarole
Glass of red wine
Fresh pineapple

D A Y   4

Breakfast
Quinoa muffins with
  raspberry preserves
Coffee with soy milk

Snack
Handful of cherries

Lunch
Soba noodles in miso soup
Green tea

Snack
Carrot-ginger juice

Dinner
Grilled red snapper
Basmati rice
Steamed artichoke
Chamomile tea
Frozen yogurt

D A Y   5

Breakfast
Kasha with brown sugar
  and soy milk
Stewed prunes
St.-John's-wort tea

Snack
Bowl of ricotta with raisins
  and cinnamon

Lunch
Peanut butter and
  blueberry jam on soy-
  flour bread
Glass of goat's milk
2 apricots

Snack
Fresh vegetables with
  tahini dip
Water with lemon

Dinner
Lasagna with rice noodles,
  spinach, ricotta, and basil
  pesto
Portobello mushrooms with
  white sauce
Romaine salad with
  mustard vinaigrette
Glass of wine
Oatmeal cookies

D A Y   6

Breakfast
Silken tofu scramble with
    peaches and blueberries
½ grapefruit
Hazelnut coffee

Snack
Fresh figs
Glass of goat's milk

Lunch
Salad pizza with whole-
    spelt crust, fresh greens,
and slivers of melted
    mozzarella
Fenugreek tea

Snack
Carrot-celery juice

Dinner
Broiled grouper with peanut
    sauce, served on a bed of
    red lentils and rice
Steamed pumpkin
Valerian tea

D A Y   7

Breakfast
Blueberry–oat bran muffin
Fresh pineapple
Cinnamon coffee

Snack
Peanuts and raisins
Glass of soy milk

Lunch
Grilled soy cheese on
    Ezekiel bread
Sliced apples and walnuts
Lemonade

Snack
Broccoli-carrot juice

Dinner
    Sesame chicken
Spelt noodles with grated
    pecorino romano cheese
Braised collard greens
Glass of red wine
Sliced mixed plums

DAY 8

Breakfast
Silken tofu scramble with
  brown rice and leftover
  collards
Ginger tea

Snack
Fruit smoothie with soy
  milk, peaches, and
  pineapple

Lunch
White bean soup with
  wilted greens and garlic

1 slice of pumpernickel
  and raisin toast
Iced fenugreek tea

Snack
Goat cheese on rye crackers
Pineapple juice

Dinner
Broiled salmon, marinated
  in tamari dipping sauce
Kasha
Stewed okra and onion
Glass of red wine

DAY 9

Breakfast
Single-egg omelet filled
  with okra and kasha,
  topped with goat cheese
Grapefruit juice
Cinnamon coffee

Snack
2 plums
Green tea

Lunch
Millet tabbouleh with
  squares of silken tofu
Iced ginger tea

Snack
Sliced apples and goat
  Cheddar

Dinner
Artichoke pasta with garlic,
  fresh spinach, walnuts,
  feta cheese, and black
  olives
Braised carrots, garlic, and
  ginger
Spelt baguette
Glass of red wine

D A Y   1 0

Breakfast
Blueberry buckwheat
  muffin
Apricot juice
Vanilla-nut coffee

Snack
Silken tofu shake with
  pineapple juice

Lunch
Lentil soup with leeks and
  carrots
Fenugreek tea

Snack
Rice cakes with soy butter
  and cherry preserves

Dinner
Cornish game hen roasted
  with onions and parsnips
Wild and basmati rice pilaf
Tossed green salad with
  mustard vinaigrette
Fresh figs
Rose hips tea

D A Y   1 1

Breakfast
Millet porridge with
  raisins, dates, sunflower
  seeds, and soy milk
Black coffee

Snack
Carrot sticks with peanut
  butter
St.-John's-wort tea

Lunch
Avocado, goat cheese,
  cucumber, and sprouts
  on sprouted-wheat bread

Pineapple juice

Snack
2 apricots
Glass of soy milk

Dinner
Grilled, marinated tempeh
Quinoa risotto
Broccoli sautéed with
  walnuts and walnut
  oil–lemon dressing
Glass of red wine
Gingerbread

DAY 12

Breakfast
1 slice of Sprouted-wheat
toast with blackberry
preserves
Coffee with soy milk

Snack
Yogurt shake with apricot
juice and peaches

Lunch
Black bean, barley, and
corn salad
Guacamole and chips
Lemonade

Snack
Carrot juice with fresh
ginger

Dinner
Portobello mushroom
burgers, topped with
mozzarella and onions, on
spelt buns
Tofu fries
Carrot-raisin salad
Glass of red wine
Watermelon slices

DAY 13

Breakfast
Oat-flour waffles with
maple syrup
Cinnamon coffee
Fresh pineapple

Snack
Walnuts and raisins
Ginseng tea

Lunch
Escarole soup with grated
pecorino romano
1 slice of whole-spelt
bread with melted soy
cheese

Glass of water with lemon

Snack
Carrot-cucumber juice

Dinner
Grilled tuna steak
Grilled zucchini, onions,
and Portobello
mushrooms
Brown rice pilaf
Dandelion and watercress
salad with mustard-lime
vinaigrette
Glass of red wine

DAY 14

Breakfast
Ezekiel French toast with
   maple syrup
Glass of pineapple juice
Coffee

Snack
½ pink grapefruit
Rose hips tea

Lunch
Grilled tuna salad
   sandwich on soy bread
Sliced apple
Water with lemon

Snack
Tamari pumpkin seeds
Iced ginger tea

Dinner
Tofu and black bean stew
Steamed rice
Glazed turnips
Romaine salad with Caesar
   dressing
Herb tea

DAY 15

Breakfast
Miso soup
Cucumber salad
Sesame seed–rice crackers
Green tea

Snack
1 slice of Essene toast with
   apricot jam
Iced coffee

Lunch
Grilled chicken salad on
   romaine with spelt
   croutons and Caesar
   dressing

Green tea

Snack
1 piece of pineapple
   upside-down cake
Hot coffee

Dinner
Spicy stir-fried tofu with
   apricots and almonds
Steamed rice
Swiss chard with garlic

D A Y   1 6

Breakfast
Millet and soy pancakes
with honey
Fresh blueberries
Grapefruit juice
Coffee

Snack
Yogurt with walnuts and
raisins
Rose hips tea

Lunch
Tofu and pumpkin
pudding
1 piece of corn bread

Snack
Fresh carrot-celery juice

Dinner
Sautéed monkfish
Whole-wheat couscous
Mesclun salad with mustard
dressing, green beans,
walnuts, and goat cheese
Glass of red wine

D A Y   1 7

Breakfast
Frittata with spinach and
feta
Fresh cherries
Vanilla-nut coffee

Snack
2 plums
Fenugreek tea

Lunch
Grilled mozzarella and
zucchini sandwich
Iced ginseng tea

Snack
Apples with walnuts and
raisins
Glass of water with lemon

Dinner
Grilled chicken breast
Brown rice pilaf
Steamed broccoli and
carrots
Ginger tea

D A Y   1 8

Breakfast
Blueberry muffins
Grapefruit juice
Cinnamon coffee

Snack
Prune-date smoothie

Lunch
Salmon salad with Rye
   Crisps
Cold artichoke with lemon
   vinaigrette
Iced ginger tea

Snack
Glass of soy milk
Pear

Dinner
Quinoa tortillas with pinto
   beans
Steamed brown rice
Romaine salad with feta and
   lemon vinaigrette
Herb tea

D A Y   1 9

Breakfast
Silken tofu scramble with
   broccoli
1 slice of Ezekiel toast
   with lemon preserves
Vanilla-nut coffee

Snack
2 plums
St.-John's-wort tea

Lunch
Black-eyed peas
1 piece of corn bread
Carrot-celery juice

Snack
Sliced apples and walnuts
Ginger tea

Dinner
Peter's Snails
Wild and basmati rice pilaf
Mesclun salad with mustard
   dressing
Glass of wine

DAY 20

Breakfast
Fresh blueberries and
  yogurt
1 slice of Ezekiel toast
  with grape jelly
Coffee

Snack
Apricot–soy milk smoothie

Lunch
Country vegetable soup
  with garlic croutons
Green tea

Snack
Soy cheese and rye crackers

Dinner
Curried lentils
Steamed amaranth
Braised dandelion greens
  with garlic
Glass of wine

DAY 21

Breakfast
Buckwheat pancakes with
  syrup
½ grapefruit
Chamomile tea

Snack
Peanut butter cookies
Coffee

Lunch
Adzuki bean and sweet
  brown rice
Small romaine salad with
  seaweed dressing

Mineral water with lemon

Snack
Toasted pumpkin seeds
Ginseng tea

Dinner
Quinoa pasta with stir-fried
  vegetables and grated
  romano
Romaine with red onions
  and lemon vinaigrette
Glass of red wine

D A Y   2 2

Breakfast
Quinoa muffins with
  raspberry jam
Fresh blackberries
Grapefruit juice
Coffee

Snack
Yogurt-pineapple smoothie

Lunch
Gingered squash soup
Rye crackers with soy
  cheese
Water with lemon

Snack
2 plums
Walnut cookies

Dinner
Tofu and curried vegetable
  stew
Brown rice
Fresh figs
Herb tea

D A Y   2 3

Breakfast
1 slice of apricot and
  almond toast with
  cherry preserves
Vanilla-nut coffee

Snack
Glass of soy milk
Carrot sticks with bean dip

Lunch
Curried tuna salad on
  Wasa crackers
Pineapple juice and water

Snack
Walnuts, raisins, and
  sunflower seeds
Green tea

Dinner
Broiled rainbow trout
Glazed root vegetables
Carrot-raisin salad
Glass of wine

D A Y   2 4

Breakfast
Single-egg omelet with
  leftover brown rice, goat
  cheese, and cilantro
Almond coffee with
  almond milk
Black cherry juice with
  water

Snack
Peeled grapefruit sections
St.-John's-wort tea

Lunch
Soy bread with ricotta,

honey, chopped walnuts,
  and raisins
Glass of pineapple juice

Snack
Tamari pumpkin seeds
Chamomile tea

Dinner
Black bean soup
Brown rice
Mesclun salad with
  mustard dressing
Pumpkin-tofu pudding

D A Y   2 5

Breakfast
Pineapple-strawberry soy
  shake

Snack
Blueberry muffin
Iced coffee

Lunch
Black-eyed pea and corn
  salad
Green salad with lemon
  vinaigrette
Carrot-celery juice

Snack
Apple with peanut butter
Green tea

Dinner
Sautéed monkfish
Wilted greens with olive oil
  and feta
Corn bread
Glass of red wine
Fresh figs

D A Y   2 6

Breakfast
Ezekiel French toast
½ grapefruit
Hot coffee with almond
 milk

Snack
Rice cakes with peanut
 butter and cherry
 preserves
St.-John's-wort tea

Lunch
Curried carrot soup
Spelt baguette
Water with lemon

Snack
Peanut butter cookies
Hot coffee

Dinner
Spinach frittata
Toasted spelt English
 muffin
Apricot, cherry, and plum
 fruit salad with yogurt
 dressing
Chamomile tea

D A Y   2 7

Breakfast
Blueberry muffin
Hot coffee with soy milk

Snack
Pineapple-yogurt shake

Lunch
Lentil soup
1 slice of Essene toast with
 melted goat Cheddar
Carrot-cucumber juice

Snack
2 plums
Ginseng tea

Dinner
Tofu with apricots and
 almonds
Steamed brown rice
Steamed broccoli
Glass of red wine

D A Y   2 8

Breakfast
Silken tofu scramble with
  sautéed apples and pears
Vanilla-nut coffee

Snack
Peach-raspberry smoothie

Lunch
Buckwheat noodles with
  peanut sauce
Green tea

Snack
Carrot-raisin salad
Ginger tea

Dinner
Grilled salmon steak with
  fresh dill
Basmati rice
Green beans with walnuts,
  goat cheese, and lemon
  vinaigrette
Glass of white wine

D A Y   2 9

Breakfast
Amaranth pancakes with
  maple syrup
Cinnamon coffee

Snack
Sliced peaches and plums
Green tea

Lunch
Pinto bean soup with leeks
  and garlic
1 slice of spelt baguette

Snack
Apple and slivers of goat
  cheese

Dinner
Tofu-vegetable stir-fry
Steamed brown rice
Walnut cookies
Ginger tea

D A Y   3 0

Breakfast
Tofu-sesame fry
Green tea

Snack
Silken tofu smoothie

Lunch
Mesclun salad topped with
    tuna salad
Fenugreek tea

Snack
Sprouted-wheat toast with
    plum preserves
Iced coffee

Dinner
Steamed red snapper with
    fresh herbs
Brown rice pilaf
Braised fennel and garlic
Glass of wine

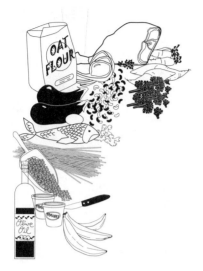

30-Day Menus for Type

B

DAY 1

Breakfast
Millet cereal with raisins,
    milk, and maple syrup
½ grapefruit
Ginger tea

Snack
Glass of kefir
Cherries

Lunch
Mashed sardines and
    lettuce on Ezekiel bread
Carrot sticks
Mineral water with lemon

Snack
Blueberry spelt muffin
Banana
Coffee

Dinner
Stuffed peppers with spelt
    berries and goat cheese
Bean salad with red onion
    and vinaigrette
Steamed cauliflower with
    lemon
Glass of red wine

D A Y   2

Breakfast
Fresh figs with goat cheese
2 slices of Ezekiel toast
   with raspberry preserves
Orange sections
Green tea

Snack
Banana-pineapple yogurt
   drink

Lunch
Gingered squash soup
Wasa bread with slice of
   cheese

Snack
Cranberry spelt muffin
2 plums
Rose hips tea

Dinner
Liver with onions
Mashed potatoes with
   butter
Grilled eggplant
Mineral water

D A Y   3

Breakfast
Single-egg omelet with
   feta cheese and chopped
   parsley
1 slice of Essene toast with
   apple butter
Papaya juice
Green tea

Snack
Apricot-yogurt drink

Lunch
Faro pilaf with goat cheese
Cucumber with oil and

vinegar
Ginseng tea

Snack
Rice cakes with almond
   butter
Grapes
Ginger tea

Dinner
Braised rabbit with orzo
Braised fennel with garlic
Tossed salad with olive oil
   and balsamic vinegar
Herb tea

DAY 4

Breakfast
Oatmeal with raisins, milk,
  and maple syrup
Pineapple juice
Coffee

Snack
Glass of soy milk
Banana

Lunch
Cherry-yogurt soup
2 plums
Ginger tea

Snack
Pear spelt muffin
Green tea

Dinner
Sautéed monkfish
Brown rice pilaf
Sautéed peppers and
  shiitake mushrooms
Glass of white wine

DAY 5

Breakfast
Ricotta with sautéed
  bananas
Papaya juice
Coffee

Snack
Slice pineapple bread
Mixed berry salad
Green tea

Lunch
Tuna salad and lettuce on
  Ezekiel bread
Carrot-cucumber juice

Snack
Walnut cookies
Orange sections
Peppermint tea

Dinner
Venison stew
Braised greens with garlic
Pan-fried sweet potatoes
Glass of red wine

DAY 6

Breakfast
1 slice of Almond-Rice
  Bread with plum
  preserves
Poached egg
½ grapefruit
Coffee

Snack
Papaya-banana yogurt
  drink

Lunch
Mixed roots soup
Grilled goat cheese
  sandwich

Snack
Lemon squares
Green tea

Dinner
Broiled halibut with
  lemongrass
Basmati rice
Steamed beets with
  vinaigrette
Tropical salad
Mineral water

DAY 7

Breakfast
Oat flour–spelt pancakes
  topped with sautéed
  pears
Grape juice
Coffee

Snack
Pineapple-yogurt
  smoothie

Lunch
Poached fruit over ricotta
Mineral water with lemon

Snack
Grapes
Green tea

Dinner
Broiled lamb chops with
  mint chutney
Brown rice
Carrots and parsnips with
  garlic, ginger, and cilantro
Sage tea

DAY 8

Breakfast
Yogurt with mixed plums
1 slice of Ezekiel bread
   with almond butter
Peppermint tea

Snack
Mango-lime soy smoothie

Lunch
Tuna salad on spelt bread
Cole slaw
Carrot-celery juice

Snack
Mixed fruit salad
Green tea

Dinner
Stuffed shells with pesto
Steamed broccoli with
   lemon
Tossed salad
Glass of wine

DAY 9

Breakfast
Single-egg omelet with
   Gruyère
1 slice of Ezekiel bread
   with butter
Pineapple juice
Coffee

Snack
Yogurt with bananas and
   raisins

Lunch
Cream of lima bean soup
Tossed salad
Mineral water with lemon

Snack
Shortbread
Grapes
Green tea

Dinner
Sautéed squid with potatoes
Steamed beet leaves with
   lemon vinaigrette
Poached pears
Glass of white wine

D A Y   1 0

Breakfast
Banana oat muffin
Papaya juice
Pineapple chunks
Coffee

Snack
Cottage cheese and grapes
Peppermint tea

Lunch
Spinach pasta with
  sautéed mushrooms and
  Parmesan

Tossed salad
Mineral water with lemon

Snack
Wasa bread with goat
  cheese
Carrot-celery juice

Dinner
Curried lamb with
  vegetables
Basmati rice
Cucumber-yogurt soup
Cardamom tea

D A Y   1 1

Breakfast
Single-egg omelet with
  feta and minced parsley
1 slice of rye bread with
  plum preserves
½ grapefruit
Green tea

Snack
Banana-yogurt smoothie

Lunch
Soft goat cheese and
  cherry preserves on
  Almond-Rice Bread

Red grapes
Mineral water with lemon

Snack
Rice pudding
2 plums
Ginger tea

Dinner
Roast turkey breast
Boiled red potatoes
Steamed beet leaves with
  raspberry vinaigrette
Glass of red wine

D A Y   1 2

Breakfast
Cream of Rice with dried
  cherries and soy-rice milk
Fresh pineapple
Coffee

Snack
Glass of kefir
Fresh papaya

Lunch
Almond butter and sliced
  bananas on Ezekiel
  bread
Grape juice

Snack
Blueberry oat muffin
Bosc pear
Green tea

Dinner
Broiled lamb chops
Millet pilaf with shiitake
  mushrooms
Braised greens with garlic
Glass of red wine

D A Y   1 3

Breakfast
Cottage cheese with fresh
  pineapple and papaya
1 slice of spelt bread with
  grape jelly
Green tea

Snack
Glass of goat's milk
Banana

Lunch
Quinoa pasta with sautéed
  mixed peppers and goat
  cheese
Mineral water

Snack
2 walnut cookies
Green grapes
Coffee

Dinner
Broiled flounder
Steamed Brussels sprouts
  with butter, lemon, and
  parsley
Brown rice
Glass of white wine

D A Y   1 4

Breakfast
Oat-spelt pancakes with
 sautéed bananas
Orange and grapefruit
 sections
Green tea

Snack
Glass of soy milk
Dried figs and dates

Lunch
Fish soup
1 slice of spelt baguette
Carrot-raisin salad

Snack
Rice crackers with goat
 cheese
Raspberry leaf tea

Dinner
Ricotta-stuffed shells with
 pesto
Braised eggplant, peppers,
 shiitake mushrooms, and
 garlic
Mesclun salad with oil and
 vinegar
Green tea

D A Y   1 5

Breakfast
Scrambled egg
2 slices of oat toast with
 orange marmalade
Pineapple juice
Green tea

Snack
Papaya-yogurt smoothie
Fresh figs

Lunch
Fresh mozzarella with
 sautéed zucchini and
 garlic on spelt baguette

Carrot celery juice

Snack
Lemon curd square
Coffee

Dinner
Turkey burger with mango
 chutney
Spelt-berry pilaf
Cole slaw
Glass of white wine

D A Y   1 6

Breakfast
Homemade granola with
  sliced bananas
Pineapple juice
Peppermint tea

Snack
Orange-yogurt smoothie
Concord grapes

Lunch
Beef burger
Cole slaw
Carrot-cucumber juice

Snack
Cranberry oat muffin
Coffee

Dinner
Broiled cod
Spinach pasta with
  cauliflower, garlic,
  and parsley
Tossed salad with feta
Glass of white wine

D A Y   1 7

Breakfast
Oatmeal with raisins,
  warm milk, and maple
  syrup
Coffee

Snack
Fruit salad
Mineral water with grape
  juice

Lunch
Grilled peppers and goat
  cheese on spelt bread
Carrot-cucumber juice

Snack
Kefir-banana smoothie
Grapes

Dinner
Indian lamb stew with
  spinach
Basmati rice
Grated cucumber and
  yogurt salad sprinkled
  with cumin seeds
Glass of white wine

D A Y   1 8

Breakfast
Miso soup
Brown rice
Salted sliced cucumbers
Green tea

Snack
Banana-pineapple smoothie

Lunch
Sardines on oat bread
Carrot-celery juice

Snack
Red grapes

Rice crackers with goat
  cheese
Ginger tea

Dinner
Grilled rainbow trout
  with butter, lemon,
  and parsley
Sweet potato fritters
Mixed sautéed peppers
  and garlic
Pineapple upside-down
  cake
Herb tea

D A Y   1 9

Breakfast
Gruyère omelet
2 slices of spelt toast with
  cherry preserves
Grapefruit juice
Green tea

Snack
Kefir and pineapple
  smoothie
Red grapes

Lunch
Kidney bean and
  butternut squash soup

Wasa bread with Monterey
  Jack cheese
Mineral water

Snack
Shortbread
Coffee

Dinner
Homemade white pizza
  with broccoli, red
  peppers, and goat
  cheese
Tossed salad
Glass of white wine

DAY 20

Breakfast
Yogurt with pineapple,
  papaya, and banana
Peppermint tea

Snack
Pear muffin
Coffee

Lunch
Curried turkey salad on
  Ezekiel bread
Mineral water with papaya
  juice

Snack
Glass of goat's milk
Dates, figs, and walnuts

Dinner
Braised rabbit
Baked sweet potato
Mango-pineapple chutney
Glass of red wine

DAY 21

Breakfast
Banana-walnut muffin
Green tea

Snack
Yogurt with honey and
  raisins
Peppermint tea

Lunch
Cream of lima bean soup
Mineral water

Snack
Handful of grapes
Ginger tea

Dinner
Broiled lamb chops with
  fresh mint sauce
Basmati rice
Mesclun salad
Glass of red wine
Oatmeal cookie

D A Y   2 2

Breakfast
Cottage cheese with sliced
  banana and honey
Cranberry tea
1 slice of spelt toast with
  plum preserves

Snack
Rice cake with soy butter
  and cherry jam
Coffee

Lunch
Apple, celery, and walnut
  salad with yogurt-honey
  dressing

Banana oat muffin
Ginger tea

Snack
Carrot-celery juice

Dinner
Pan-fried monkfish
Roasted new potatoes with
  garlic and rosemary
½ baked acorn squash with
  butter and honey
Wilted mustard greens
  with garlic
Mineral water

D A Y   2 3

Breakfast
Pineapple-yogurt shake
Green tea

Snack
1 slice of pineapple bread
Espresso

Lunch
Simple fish soup
Carrot-raisin salad
Ginger tea

Snack
Sliced red and yellow
  peppers with curry dip
Mineral water

Dinner
Indian lamb stew with
  spinach
Brown rice pilaf
Fresh sliced mango and
  peaches
Rose water lassi

DAY 24

Breakfast
Millet-spelt-soy pancakes
  with maple syrup
Vanilla-nut coffee with
  milk

Snack
Banana-peach yogurt
  shake

Lunch
Tuna melt on spelt bread
  with lettuce and tomato
Mineral water with lemon

Snack
Carrot-ginger juice

Dinner
Green green pasta
Grilled lamb sausages
Glass of white wine

DAY 25

Breakfast
Single-egg omelet with
  broccoli and cheddar
Cappuccino
Mineral water

Snack
Yogurt
Handful of grapes

Lunch
Alder-smoked mackerel
  salad on spelt bread
Romaine salad with feta
Iced herbal tea

Snack
Goat cheese and apple
Mineral water

Dinner
Yankee pot roast
Spelt French bread
Green bean salad
Poached fruit
Glass of red wine

DAY 26

Breakfast
Puffed rice cereal with
  milk and bananas
Black coffee

Snack
Dried apricots and papaya
St.-John's-wort tea

Lunch
Cucumber-yogurt soup
Banana-plum cake
Green tea

Snack
Rice cake with almond
  butter and grape jelly
Rose hips tea

Dinner
Broiled sole
Roasted potatoes with garlic
Sautéed broccoli rabe and
  onions
Glass of white wine

DAY 27

Breakfast
Apricot-yogurt shake
1 slice of raisin toast with
  butter
Coffee

Snack
Carrot sticks with dill
  cottage cheese dip
Peppermint tea

Lunch
Lima bean salad with goat
  cheese
Fresh figs

Mineral water with lemon

Snack
  Hot turkey broth

Dinner
  Venison stew
  Sautéed apples and pears
    with raisins
  2 slices of spelt French
    bread
  Gruyère cheese
  Herbal tea

D A Y   2 8

Breakfast
French toast with maple
   syrup
Sliced banana
Cappuccino

Snack
Rose hips tea

Lunch
Cottage cheese with grated
   carrots and jicama on
   romaine with balsamic
   honey-mustard dressing
Mineral water with lemon

Snack
Apricots and almonds
Green tea

Dinner
Grilled flank steak
Grilled red and yellow
   peppers and zucchini
Brown rice pilaf
Glass of red wine

D A Y   2 9

Breakfast
Single-egg omelet with
   leftover grilled
   vegetables and
   goat cheese
Papaya juice
Green tea

Snack
Pineapple-yogurt smoothie

Lunch
Greek salad
Spelt roll
Ginseng tea

Snack
Cranberry juice
2 oatmeal cookies

Dinner
Roast turkey
Sweet potato purée
Cranberry dressing
Green beans with balsamic
   vinaigrette
Mineral water

D A Y   3 0

Breakfast
Hot oatmeal with milk and
  dried cherries
Coffee

Snack
Papaya smoothie

Lunch
Turkey soup
Spelt French bread
Ginger tea

Snack
Apple with Cheddar cheese
Rose hips tea

Dinner
Grilled lamb chops
Grilled eggplant and red
  peppers with goat cheese
Green salad with lemon and
  olive oil dressing
Glass of wine

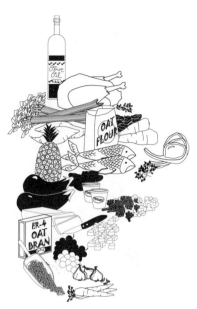

30-Day Menus for Type

AB

D A Y 1

Breakfast
Wild rice pudding
Grapes
Coffee

Snack
Papaya-kiwi soy shake

Lunch
Peanut butter, raisins, and
honey on Ezekiel bread
Cranberry juice

Snack
Pineapple spelt muffin
Green tea

Dinner
Fried monkfish over pasta
with parsley
Steamed broccoli with
lemon
Sliced tomatoes, red onion,
and lemon vinaigrette

D A Y   2

Breakfast
Single-egg omelet with
    mozzarella and leftover
    steamed broccoli
Carrot juice
Green tea

Snack
Apricot lassi

Lunch
Onion soup with French
    bread and Gruyère
Tossed salad

Snack
Lemon bread
Cherries
Coffee

Dinner
Grilled curried leg of lamb
Basmati rice
Braised greens
Cucumber salad
Green tea

D A Y   3

Breakfast
Spelt pancakes with
    sautéed apples
Papaya juice
½ grapefruit
Coffee

Snack
Pinapple-kiwi yogurt
    shake

Lunch
Lentil soup
Tossed salad
Mineral water with lemon

Snack
Wasa bread with goat
    cheese
Cherries
Green tea

Dinner
Salmon with garlic, ginger,
    and cilantro
Brown rice
Braised celery
Glass of white wine

DAY 4

Breakfast
Cottage cheese with fresh
  pineapple and kiwi
1 slice of soy bread with
  cherry preserves
Coffee

Snack
Blueberry oat muffin
Ginger tea

Lunch
Turkey soup
Rye bread with sliced goat
  cheese

Snack
Kefir
Mixed plums

Dinner
Grilled rainbow trout
Mashed sweet potatoes
Grilled eggplant and
  zucchini
Glass of white wine
Grapes

DAY 5

Breakfast
Oatmeal with dried
  cranberries, maple syrup,
  and goat milk
Pineapple juice
Coffee

Snack
Glass of soy milk
Grapes

Lunch
Tuna salad with
  mayonnaise and alfalfa
  sprouts on rye bread

Carrot and celery sticks
Mineral water with lemon

Snack
Blueberry spelt muffin
Apple
Green tea

Dinner
Liver with mushrooms
  and onions
Roasted new potatoes with
  herbs
Braised dandelion greens
  with garlic
Glass of wine

D A Y   6

Breakfast
Single-egg omelet with
   feta, tomato, and basil
I slice of Almond-Rice
   Bread with apricot
   preserves
½ grapefruit
Coffee

Snack
Yogurt with sliced kiwi
Green tea

Lunch
Pinto bean chili
Brown rice

Mixed salad

Snack
I slice of pineapple bread
Cherries
Ginger tea

Dinner
Poached red snapper
Spinach pasta with
   cauliflower and garlic
Sliced tomatoes,
   cucumbers, and red
   onion with lemon
   vinaigrette

D A Y   7

Breakfast
Millet cereal with raisins
   and soy milk
½ grapefruit
Coffee

Snack
Handful of peanuts,
   walnuts, and chocolate
   chips
Pear

Lunch
Bean salad with red onion,
   goat cheese, and lemon
   vinaigrette

Mineral water

Snack
Baklava
Coffee

Dinner
Rabbit stew with carrots,
   potatoes, celery, and
   parsnips
Braised spinach with garlic
French bread
Tropical fruit salad

DAY 8

Breakfast
Yogurt with honey, walnut,
   and raisins
Grapefruit sections
Green tea

Snack
Cottage cheese with
   pineapple
Rose hips tea

Lunch
Sardines with lemon
   squeeze on rye bread
Carrot-celery juice

Snack
Peanut butter cookies
Peach and apricots

Dinner
Turkey breast with
   pineapple chutney
Wild rice salad with walnuts
Boiled, mashed plantains
Glass of white wine

DAY 9

Breakfast
2 poached eggs
Fresh figs with goat cheese
1 slice of sprouted-wheat
   toast with grapefruit
   marmalade
Green tea

Snack
Glass of soy-rice milk
Apple

Lunch
Stewed fruit on ricotta
Papaya juice

Snack
Spelt-bread pudding
Coffee

Dinner
Tuna steak with cherry
   tomatoes
Brown basmati rice
Braised turnips
Wilted greens salad with
   goat cheese
Mineral water

D A Y   1 0

Breakfast
Citrus salad
Pineapple juice
Ginger tea

Snack
Date-prune shake

Lunch
Spelt berry salad with
    cucumber, parsley, and
    feta cheese
Carrot-celery juice

Snack
Peanut butter on rice
    crackers
Grapes
Coffee

Dinner
Grilled marinated tempeh
Eggplant garlic stew
Steamed quinoa
Halved red and yellow
    cherry tomatoes with
    lemon vinaigrette

D A Y   1 1

Breakfast
Spelt-bread pudding
Grapes
Coffee

Snack
Glass of goat's milk
Cherries and pineapple

Lunch
Miso soup with tofu
Brown rice
Cucumber salad

Snack
Peanut butter candy
Green tea

Dinner
Broiled lamb chops
Mashed sweet potatoes
Braised cauliflower with
    garlic

DAY 12

Breakfast
Citrus salad
Grapefruit juice
Coffee

Snack
Yogurt with fresh kiwis
Mineral water

Lunch
Pinto bean salad with
  garlic dressing
Celery-carrot juice
Rye crackers with sheep
  cheese

Snack
Pumpkin bread with
  walnuts
Coffee

Dinner
Grouper with peanut crust
Basmati rice
Braised dandelion greens
  with garlic
Glass of white wine
Plum cake

DAY 13

Breakfast
Scrambled egg
2 slices of turkey bacon
2 slices of oat toast with
  grapefruit marmalade
Green tea

Snack
Glass of soy milk
Green grapes

Lunch
Tuna salad on rye bread
  with alfalfa sprouts
Carrot-celery juice

Snack
Fruit salad with peanut
  dressing
Ginsing tea

Dinner
Lasagna with Portobello
  mushrooms and pesto
Tossed salad with lemon
  vinaigrette
Spelt baguette
Glass of red wine

D A Y 1 4

Breakfast
Oat-spelt pancakes with
    maple syrup
½ grapefruit
Coffee

Snack
Yogurt with walnuts,
    raisins, and honey drizzle
Ginger tea

Lunch
Lentil salad with sheep
    cheese
Mineral water

Snack
Cherry muffin
Green tea

Dinner
Rabbit stew
Braised greens with garlic
1 slice of pear cake
Glass of red wine

D A Y 1 5

Breakfast
Oatmeal with warm milk,
    dried cherries, and
    maple syrup
Green tea

Snack
Ricotta with fresh
    pineapple
Cranberry juice

Lunch
Basmati and wild rice salad
    with tofu and parsley
    pesto

Carrot-cucumber juice

Snack
Gingerbread
Coffee

Dinner
Red snapper
Spelt pilaf
Steamed beets with butter
    and lemon
Poached fruit
Herbal ice tea

DAY 16

Breakfast
½ grapefruit
Fresh figs with goat cheese
Oat-bran muffin
Green tea

Snack
Yogurt-pineapple smoothie

Lunch
Cream of broccoli soup
1 slice of spelt baguette
  with sheep cheese
Mineral water

Snack
Peanut butter and cherry
  preserves on Wasa bread
Green tea

Dinner
Lamb kabobs
Sweet potato salad
Wilted greens with ricotta
  salata
Glass of red wine

DAY 17

Breakfast
Omelet with feta and
  wilted greens
1 slice of rye toast with
  butter
Grapefruit juice
Coffee

Snack
Ricotta with walnuts, dates,
  and honey-lemon
  dressing
Rose hips tea

Lunch
Sardines with alfalfa

sprouts on rye bread
Carrot-celery juice

Snack
Peanut butter cookies
Coffee

Dinner
Tofu and curried vegetable
  stew
Brown rice
Cucumber and young
  dandelion greens with oil
  and lemon
Green tea

D A Y   1 8

Breakfast
Hot millet with raisins,
    warm milk, and honey
Coffee

Snack
Glass of soy milk
Peach and a plum

Lunch
Lentil soup
1 slice of baguette with
    sheep cheese
Mineral water

Snack
1 slice of lemon-walnut
    cake
Coffee

Dinner
Turkey loaf
Boiled red potatoes
Braised celery
Glass of white wine

D A Y   1 9

Breakfast
Homemade granola with
    raisins and soy milk
½ grapefruit
Coffee

Snack
Cottage cheese with fresh
    pineapple
Grape juice

Lunch
Tofu-vegetable fry
Brown rice
Cucumber salad with red
    onion

Snack
Rye Crisps with sheep
    cheese
Concord grapes

Dinner
Steamed red snapper with
    dipping sauce
Quinoa with cilantro pesto
Puréed parsnips
Glass of white wine

DAY 20

Breakfast
Omelet with soy cheese
2 slices of Ezekiel toast
  with plum preserves
Grapefruit juice
Coffee

Snack
Glass of kefir
Black grapes

Lunch
Gigered squash soup
Rye Crisps with goat
  cheese
Mineral water with lemon

Snack
2 walnut cookies
Pear
Green tea

Dinner
Curried lamb stew
Basmati rice
Cucumber-yogurt soup
Ginger tea

DAY 21

Breakfast
Yogurt with honey,
  walnuts, and raisins
Grapefruit sections
Coffee and steamed milk

Snack
Pineappple-kiwi smoothie

Lunch
Spelt berry salad with feta,
  cucumber, and scallions
Green tea

Snack
Peanut butter on apple
  slices
Glass of mineral water

Dinner
Tofu and curried vegetable
  stew
Brown rice
Pear and walnut salad
Glass of wine

D A Y   2 2

Breakfast
Millet-spelt-soy pancakes
  with maple syrup
Cranberry juice
Coffee

Snack
Glass of goat's milk
Grapes

Lunch
Grilled Portobello
  mushroom burger on a
  spelt English muffin
Seltzer with grape juice

Snack
Trail mix
Ginger tea

Dinner
Roast turkey with
  chestnut–spelt bread
  stuffing
Cranberry dressing
Mashed potatoes with skins
Glazed turnips and parsnips
Steamed greens
Mineral water

D A Y   2 3

Breakfast
Hot oatmeal with raisins
  and soy milk
Coffee

Snack
Glass of kefir
Fresh pineapple and
  strawberries

Lunch
Gingered squash soup
Sprouted-wheat toast
Glass of apple juice

Snack
Rye Crisps and goat cheese
Sliced pear
Green tea

Dinner
Fettuccine with lamb
  sausages and vegetables
Green salad
Glass of red wine

D A Y 2 4

Breakfast
Silken tofu scramble with
blueberries
Macadamia nut coffee

Snack
Oat-bran muffin with
cherry preserves
Rose hips tea

Lunch
Turkey salad on rye with
tomato and lettuce
Iced chamomile tea

Snack
Carrot-ginger juice

Dinner
Pan-fried grouper
Steamed brown rice
Sesame broccoli
Green salad with crumbled
goat cheese
Herbal ice tea

D A Y 2 5

Breakfast
Whole-wheat bagel with
cream cheese and fig
preserves
Coffee

Snack
Grape-peach yogurt shake

Lunch
Greek salad
1 slice of spelt baguette
Mineral water with lemon

Snack
2 plums
Iced ginger tea

Dinner
Turkey noodle soup
Pan-fried eggplant and
sliced tomato with goat
cheese and basil
Glass of wine

D A Y   2 6

Breakfast
Puffed-rice cereal with
  dried cherries and goat's
  milk
½ honeydew melon
Green tea

Snack
1 slice of lemon tea cake
Coffee

Lunch
White bean soup with
  wilted Swiss chard

Rye crackers with Gruyère
Mineral water with lime

Snack
Oat bran–cherry muffin
Peppermint tea

Dinner
Grilled curried leg of lamb
  with fresh mint sauce
Grilled sweet potatoes
Wild rice and basmati pilaf
Arugula salad with feta

D A Y   2 7

Breakfast
Cottage cheese with
  pineapple
1 slice of sprouted-wheat
  toast with grapefruit
  marmalade
Coffee

Snack
Miso soup with tofu

Lunch
Tuna salad sandwich on
  spelt bread with sliced
  tomato and lettuce

Iced ginger tea

Snack
Carrot-celery juice

Dinner
Turkey pot pie
Mesclun salad with olive oil
  and lemon dressing
Pineapple upside-down
  cake
Herbal tea

DAY 28

Breakfast
Single-egg omelet with
broccoli and goat
Cheddar
½ grapefruit
Cinnamon coffee

Snack
Apple and walnuts
Echinacea tea

Lunch
Sliced curried lamb on
greens with pineapple-
yogurt dressing

Grapes
Ginger tea

Snack
Fin Crisp with goat cheese
Carrot-cucumber juice

Dinner
Steamed red snapper with
seaweed dressing
Vegetable fritters
Braised fennel and garlic
Glass of wine
Poached pears

DAY 29

Breakfast
Silken tofu scramble with
sautéed pears
Coffee with steamed milk

Snack
Yogurt with honey,
walnuts, and raisins
Ginseng tea

Lunch
Curried red lentil soup
I slice of spelt bread with
goat cheese
Black cherry juice

Snack
Roasted chestnuts and
dates
Strawberry leaf tea

Dinner
Boiled tempeh with peanut
sauce
Wild and basmati rice pilaf
Steamed broccoli and
cauliflower with garlic
and parsley

D A Y   3 0

Breakfast
Peanut butter and grape
  jelly on sprouted wheat
  bread
Coffee

Snack
Fruit salad of kiwi, grapes,
  and pineapple with
  ricotta-honey dressing
Chamomile tea

Lunch
Thick fish soup
Seltzer with cranberry juice

Snack
Yogurt with sliced plums
Green tea

Dinner
Indian lamb stew with
  spinach
Pineapple chutney
Marinated cucumbers
Brown rice
Rose water lassi
Walnut cookies

Mail-Order
Marketplace

ORGANIZATION/ COMPANY	PRODUCT LINE	ADDRESS/PHONE NUMBER
The Coach Farm Inc.	Goat Products	105 Mill Hill Road Pine Plains, NY 12567 518-398-5325
Horizon Organic Dairy	Dairy Products	P.O. Box 17577 Boulder, CO 80308 1-888-494-3020
Juniper Valley Farms	Dairy Products	155-04 Liberty Avenue Jamaica, NY 11433 718-291-3333
Seven Stars Farms	Yogurt	501 West Seven Stars Road Phoenixville, PA 19460 610-935-1949
Stony Field Farm	Yogurt	10 Burton Drive Londonderry, NH 03053 603-437-4040
Coleman Natural Products, Inc.	Organic Meats	5140 Race Court Denver, CO 80216 1-800-442-8666
D'Artagnan	Specialty Meat & Poultry	280 Wilson Avenue Newark, NJ 07105 973-344-0565
Ebberley Poultry Inc.	Organic Poultry	1095 Mt. Airy Road Stevens, PA 17578 717-336-6440

ORGANIZATION/ COMPANY	PRODUCT LINE	ADDRESS/PHONE NUMBER
Murray's Free Roaming Chicken	Free-Range Chicken	334 Main Street South Fallsburg, NY 12779 914-436-5001
North American Pharmacal, Inc.	Blood Type Specialty Products	17 High Street Norwalk, CT 06851 203-866-7664
Pavich Family Farms	Dried Fruit & Nuts	P.O. Box 10420 Terra Bella, CA 93270 209-782-8700
Annie's Homegrown	Pasta Products	395 Main Street Wakefield, MA 01880 781-224-1172
Diamond Organics	Vegetables, Fruits, Nuts	P.O. Box 2159 Freedom, CA 95019 1-888-674-2642
Purity Foods	Spelt Flour & Pastas	2871 West Jolly Road Okemos, MI 48864 517-351-9231
Walnut Acres Organic Farms	Large Volume of Organic Products	Walnut Acres Road Penns Creek, PA 17862 717-837-0601

Local food co-ops carry both groceries and fresh produce.

Local health-food stores and their owner/employees are good resources for specific products.

MISCELLANEOUS

Menominee Paper Co.	Natural Wax Paper Made from Unbleached Fibers	144 First Street Menominee, MI 49858 906-863-5595
Harmony c/o Giaim Inc.	Natural Paper Products	360 Interlocken Boulevard Broomfield, CO 80021 1-800-456-1177

Join the
Blood Type Web

www.dadamo.com

THE WORLD WIDE WEB HAS PROVEN TO BE A VALUABLE venue for exploring and applying the tenets of the Blood Type Diet. Since January 1997, more than 575,000 have visited the site to participate in the ABO chat groups, to peruse the scientific archives, to share experiences and recipes, and to learn more about the science of blood type.

One of the most important features on the Web page is the Blood Type Outcome Registry, which has facilitated the collection of data on the measurable effects of the Blood Type Diet on a wide range of medical conditions.

I invite you to share your outcome, either at the Web site or by filling out the form below and sending it to:

Blood Type Outcome Registry
P.O. Box 2106
Norwalk, CT 06852-2106

Blood Type Outcome Registry

I APPRECIATE your taking the time to answer these questions about experiences you have had with the program. Your feedback can be critical in showing indicators and trends which can then be further studied. All information supplied on this form will be held in complete confidence.

Name: _____

Your Blood Type: ____ Type O ____ Type A ____ Type B ____ Type AB

How old are you? _____

Your gender: ____ Female ____ Male

Was your condition: ____ Worsened ____ No Change ____ Improved

How would you rate this degree of change? _____

_____

What health category did you see the change in? _____

_____

How long did you follow the diet before noticing changes? _____

_____

Comments and specifics: _____

_____

_____

_____

_____

_____

_____

Has this been verified clinically (lab result, etc.)? _____

_____

May we contact you about your experience? _____

Address: _____

City: _____ State: _____ Zip: _____

Phone: _____ e-mail: _____

Quick & Easy
At-Home
Blood Type Test
and
Blood Type
Specialty Products

NORTH AMERICAN PHARMACAL, INC., IS THE OFFICIAL distributor of the Home Blood Type Kits and Blood Type Specialty Products. The product line includes supplements, books, audiotapes, a bi-monthly newsletter, meal replacement bars, protein powders and support materials that make "eating right for your type" easier to incorporate into your life. One of the most popular items North American Pharmacal distributes is the At-Home Blood Type Kit which allows you to find out your blood type in five minutes. Each single-use kit is $10.75 plus $4.25 shipping and handling.

Product information and price lists are available from:

North American Pharmacal, Inc.
17 High Street
Norwalk, CT 06851
TEL: 203-866-7664
FAX: 203-838-4066

Or, if you prefer, you can contact the company through the Web site at www.dadamo.com.

Index